ADMIT ONE

What You MUST Know When Going to the Hospital

BUT NO ONE ACTUALLY TELLS YOU!

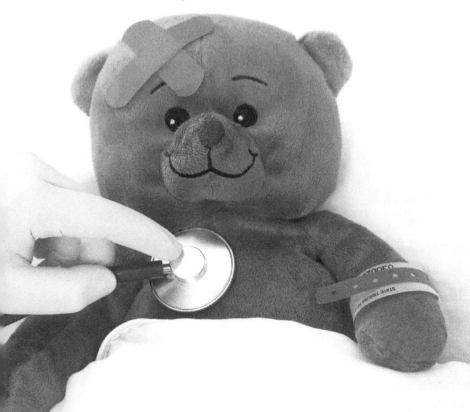

KATI KLEBER, BSN, RN, CCRN

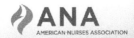

ANA
AMERICAN NURSES ASSOCIATION

American Nurses Association
8515 Georgia Avenue, Suite 400
Silver Spring, MD 20910-3492
1-800-274-4ANA
http://www.Nursingworld.org

American Nurses Association

The American Nurses Association (ANA) is the premier organization representing the interests of the nation's 3.4 million registered nurses. ANA advances the nursing profession by fostering high standards of nursing practice, promoting a safe and ethical work environment, bolstering the health and wellness of nurses, and advocating on health care issues that affect nurses and the public. ANA is at the forefront of improving the quality of health care for all.

Cataloging-in-Publication Data on file with the Library of Congress.

ISBN-13: 978-1-55810-655-0   SAN: 851-3481

1.0K   05/2016

First printing: May 2016.

CONTENTS

AUTHOR'S INTRODUCTION: INSIDER INFO

Hello there! Let me take a moment to introduce myself. My name is Kati and I am a nationally certified registered critical care nurse in Charlotte, North Carolina.

I have been a nurse for six years. I worked in a cardiac step-down unit for two years and have been working in a neurosciences intensive care unit for the last four years. I have my Bachelor of Science in Nursing (BSN) and am a nationally certified critical care nurse. In addition to being a bedside nurse, I am also the author of the popular nursing blog, NurseEyeRoll.com, and two additional books entitled *Becoming Nursey: From Code Blues to Code Browns, How to Care for Your Patients and Yourself* (2014), and *Now What??? The Smart Nurse's Guide to Your Dream Job* (2016).

As a nurse, I have noticed that there are quite a few things that we, as the health care team, assume you know. However, having experience as a patient myself, I have noticed that no one tells actually you these things along the way! Like many of you, I have also had family members and loved ones walk through the medical system who have come up with questions and confusion. The content in this book was compiled from my experiences to fill that gap.

What kinds of things am I talking about? I'm talking about the difference between a resident, a medical student, an attending physician, and a consulting physician. I'm talking about the difference between a physical therapist and an occupational therapist, or how physician's schedules work. We're getting down to the nitty-gritty here!

The fact that these questions are left unanswered, assuming that everyone is aware, has left me feeling like we could do a better job of informing our patients of what to expect. While it may be basic information to those of us working in the hospital day in and day out, we realize that it may not be so obvious to everyone else. The only reason it is basic information to the health care team is because we live and breathe it every day, and sometimes I think we forget that our patients do not. You have the right to not only know these things, but also to fully understand them to allow yourself and your loved ones to make the best decisions possible about your health.

HOW I LEARNED WHAT I WRITE

The information contained in this book is from my personal experiences working with patients since 2007. I have worked in the capacity of a certified nurse's assistant, nursing student, nursing intern, and finally as a registered nurse on various nursing units. I have worked in a nursing home and on critical care units. I've had experience as a nurse in many settings, from schools alongside the school nurse, to prisons, mental health facilities, and emergency departments, and worked intermediate units and nursing floors. While my experience has been mainly in large acute care hospitals, most of this information can also be applied to smaller community hospitals. However, please keep in mind that their processes may differ from those explained in this book.

My goal is to help you understand the culture of a hospital as quickly as possible, so that you can make informed decisions about your health care, know what we expect of you, and what you can expect of us. Hospital culture can be a difficult thing to understand when you are being rushed from place to place. It is a fast-paced environment with many different people filling many different roles. While all of these are necessary, it can be difficult to know who everyone is and why they are walking into your hospital room.

I want to help you know what to anticipate during your stay so that you can navigate the system with ease and feel like a pro. By reading the information contained in this book, I hope to eliminate some of the unknown and answer some of the questions you may have about how things work, as well as what your health care team expects from you and what you can expect from your health care team. It is important for you to focus on healing and by removing doubt and providing reassurance, I hope to enable you to do so.

You are the reason we are here, the reason we love coming to work every day, and the reason why we want to continue to care for patients for decades to come. We are all on one team with you at the center.

HOW TO USE THIS BOOK

Once you start reading, you'll notice I address *you* frequently. As an author, I am addressing you as a patient or someone about to become a patient in a hospital. However, you could also be reading the book with or on the behalf of a loved one—a spouse, a child, a parent, another family member, a close partner, or a good friend. (Throughout most nursing, the term *patient* by definition often includes both the patient and their support system: the people near and dear to the patient.) So just swap in *you and your [...]* any place I'm addressing you directly, and that's who I am talking to.

I also frequently use *we* to describe the health care team, as if I were a member of your health care team, speaking on behalf of your nurse.

This book is meant to help you navigate through a hospital admission. There may be some sections that apply to you or your loved ones and some that do not during this admission. There is no need to read cover-to-cover, start to finish. Please feel free to see which chapters are important and necessary for you or your loved ones.

At the end of the book there are pages left for you to take notes when your health care team rounds and gives you new information. You will notice the term "rounds" used frequently. This refers to when a member of your health care team comes to see you while you are in the hospital, speak with you, and update the plan of care. A lot of information is discussed quickly and this will provide a centralized place for you to take notes during these rounds and write down questions you think of throughout the day, as well as the answers once you receive them.

Avoiding information overload when possible is essential when in the hospital, therefore read what is important and forego what does not apply, taking notes as needed. Keep in mind, too, topics that are not applicable during this admission may become important in the future.

ACKNOWLEDGMENTS

I would like to thank my God, my husband, my family, and my colleagues. I thank God for His blessing and grace. I thank my husband and family for their constant encouragement, love, support, and honesty. I thank my colleagues for their input, experience, and the care they give their patients. I would also like to thank each and every patient and their loved ones that I've had the honor of caring for over the years, who have opened my eyes to the educational needs that come with a hospital admission. I pray the information in this book will enable patients and families to feel like a knowledgeable part of the health care team and enlighten students who are interested in being a part of the team.

SECTION 1
BEFORE YOUR STAY: MEET YOUR HEALTH CARE TEAM

This section describes all of the people who will or might come see you during your hospital stay. Each person has her or his own skills and expertise to be a part of the team of amazing professionals who will be caring for you. I will discuss most, but not all, members of this team, including some details of the educational requirements for their roles.

Here's what you can learn about in this section:

▷ The nurses and others who are on the nursing team

▷ What hospital nurses do for their patients

▷ The doctors and others who are on the medical team, including medical and surgical specialists

▷ The therapy services team, including physical therapists, occupational therapists, respiratory therapists, and speech therapists

▷ The rest of the team: pharmacists, dieticians, chaplains, social workers, case managers, unit secretaries...and your family, loved ones, and (I hope) visitors

Charge nurse: A nurse designated to be in charge of the flow of a *nursing unit* (see below), address issues that may arise, assign nurses to care for incoming patients, and work closely with management throughout each shift.

Clinical: Refers to (1) treatment given in a medical facility (for example, a hospital) or a situation requiring a medical treatment, or (2) an experience of health care providers in a health care setting (for example, a nursing student completing their clinicals).

Facility: A building in which medical evaluation and treatment occur.

Nurse manager: A nurse that manages the employees and patients of a specific nursing unit. Nurse managers typically do not care for patients directly, but work in an administrative capacity.

Primary care doctor: The doctor who you see for at least your yearly physical in your routine-care clinical setting and who refers you to other doctors and health care professionals.

Unit (nursing unit): A group of hospital rooms in one location with its own team of nurses trained to care for specific patient populations.

THE NURSING TEAM: NURSES AND OTHERS

The first group of people that I am going to speak in-depth about is the nursing team. This includes the specific nurse assigned to your care on a given shift, as well as the other nurses, nursing assistants, and other unlicensed staff members on your unit.

The Nurses: General and Specialty Practitioners

Every patient in the hospital will have a nurse who is responsible for coordinating every aspect of his or her care. Nurses can have an associate's degree in nursing (ADN) which is a two-year degree, or a bachelor's degree in nursing (BSN). Most nurses who do have a master's or doctorate degree in nursing do not work at the bedside providing direct patient care, but there are some. Most master's- or doctorate-prepared nurses work in leadership, management, education, or research. Nurses caring for patients within the health care team work to complete various tasks, provide education, and coordinate your care.

Nurses can also become certified in their specialty. They are then referred to as "nationally certified nurses" or "certified nurses." To become certified, you must work within your specialty for a minimum amount of time, specified by each nursing *specialty* (typically two years) and pass a rigorous exam. Passing this exam and becoming certified allows nurses to add credentials following her or his name on paperwork and hospital badges. These letters abbreviate the nursing *credential*, which testifies that a nurse has skills and knowledge in a given specialty.

For example, my credentials are Kati Kleber, BSN, RN, CCRN. That means I am a bachelor's-prepared (BSN) registered nurse (RN) who is a nationally certified critical care nurse (CCRN). Any nurse who is nationally certified is usually very proud of such an accomplishment! Nurses can have more than one certification, as some are applicable to multiple areas. For example, your emergency department nurse can be certified in critical care and emergency nursing, as well as a few others, because of how different their patient population can be.

What difference does it make to you as a patient whether a nurse has two years or four years of education? While they have a different degree and different credentials, when they are working at the bedside, it does not change their scope of practice. The ADN nurse can do anything the BSN nurse can, and vice versa. The current trend in nursing is for all nurses to eventually obtain their BSN degree.

Types of nursing education

▶ Associate's degree in nursing (ADN): This degree allows nurses to work at the bedside in as little as two years. The coursework and clinical work is very quick, vigorous, and challenging, as they must pass the same licensing exam as the BSN-prepared nurse but have significantly less time.

▶ Bachelor of Science in Nursing (BSN): This degree takes longer, but the trend in nursing education is for all nurses to eventually obtain this degree. The coursework can cover topics ranging from clinical, scientific, and technical subjects to professional nursing issues such as ethics and nursing practice standards.

Types of nursing certification

Nationally recognized certification is typically indicated on the nurse's badge or with a pin. There are many different certifications for many specialties, and they are accredited through the American Nurses Credentialing Center (ANCC) or another credentialing center.

During your stay you may also encounter nurses who have a graduate degree. Below is the list of the four different advanced practice registered nurses (APRNs) that you may encounter:

▸ *Nurse Practitioners (NPs):* This APRN is different from a regular RN in that they can diagnose and treat illnesses. NPs can specialize in many different areas from cardiology, to psychiatry, to emergency medicine, to neurology. They typically work closely with a particular physician or group of physicians but can also function independently.

▸ *Certified Registered Nurse Anesthetists (CRNAs):* These APRNs specialize in the administration of anesthesia. They frequently work closely with anesthesiologists.

▸ *Certified Nurse Midwives (CNMs):* CNMs care for pregnant patients, deliver babies, and can care for patients in the postpartum period as well. Many times, they work closely with the obstetrics and gynecological physicians.

▸ *Clinical Nurse Specialists (CNSs):* This group of APRNs occasionally work directly with patients, but many times work to educate the nursing staff to improve outcomes and provide expertise on a larger scale.

Your Nurse's Top Priority

Yes, there are many types of nurses in a hospital. By far, the most important thing to any of your nurses is your safety. While you are in the hospital, the environment is very different from home. Your routine is off. Your sleep is interrupted. Maybe you have had a procedure or surgery that compromised your ability to walk around normally. People become confused easily, forget where they are, and overestimate their abilities to get up and walk around, which makes them a much higher risk to fall and cause further injury. This is why safety is our top priority. Therefore, we do a lot of things to make sure you are safe. Some things may seem silly, like wearing a wrist band that says "fall risk" or someone walking with you to the bathroom every time you go, but they are a very important part of your care.

Nursing Reports, Schedules, and Staffing

Most nurses work 12-hour shifts three days per week. Most 12-hour shifts begin around 7:00 a.m. and end around 7:00 p.m., although there are some hospitals and units that do this differently. Our shifts overlap so that we can share important information about the patients. One of the wonderful things about most nurses working 12 hours at a time is that you will have only two different nurses in a 24-hour period. If a nurse is working a few days in a row, most will try to accommodate it so that you have the same nurse. It's always nice to have a familiar face and someone who knows you well.

Most hospitals assign patients to nurses based on their location in the unit (meaning a block of patient rooms goes to one nurse), how sick they are or how complex their care is (acuity), or a combination of both. Not all patients are created equal. Some will require more time and attention than others depending on their needs, and therefore we must assign the staff where they are needed. This can mean that your nurse may change in the middle of the day to better accommodate this. Patient safety is the name of the game! If one nurse has all of the sickest patients, requiring the most intense care, it will not allow him or her to give each patient the care they deserve and require. This is why you may or may not get the same nurse two to three days in a row.

If you are in an intensive care unit, nurses are typically only responsible for one to two patients each. If you're in a step-down or intermediate unit, nurses are usually taking care of three to four patients each. If you're on a regular nursing unit, nurses can be responsible for coordinating the care of anywhere from four to seven patients each. I will discuss the differences in units later. Please keep in mind that this does differ across hospitals.

Report and Shift Change of Nurses

Between each shift, something called "report" occurs, which really means: The offgoing nurse and the oncoming nurse talk about you! They talk about what brought you to the hospital, your medical–surgical history, your plan of care, your lab values, and many other things. Report usually lasts approximately 30 minutes for the oncoming nurse to get information on his or her entire "patient load" (patient load meaning all of the patients they will be responsible for during this shift). This information sharing session is fast-paced. Your oncoming nurse is learning all about you and it is essential they focus. It can be a bit of a chaotic time while the entire unit is sharing information and changing shifts.

Many facilities have implemented "bedside reporting," meaning that instead of occurring in the nurse's station or hallway, report occurs at your bedside so you can participate, interject, and correct information if needed.

> **PATIENT TIP!**   If you're a loved one or family member, I recommend not calling the unit for an update during shift change/report. You will either talk to a nurse who's been working for 12 hours straight or one who is just learning your loved one's name. I would wait 1 to 2 hours after report, that way your new nurse has a chance to dive into the chart, introduce themselves, and talk to the rest of the health care team to coordinate the day.
>
> I'm not saying never call at this time (if this is the best time for you then do what you need to do!), but if it can be helped, I would wait until after this occurs—you will get a much better and more detailed update!

Responsibilities of Nurses

Your nurse is responsible for many different things. They work closely with the health care team to discuss everything about your care. They work with your rehab services (physical therapist, occupational therapist, and/or speech therapist), case manager, pharmacist, social worker, dietician/nutritionist, chaplain, and anyone else who takes part in your care. The nurse is the coordinator of all of these different people.

One main responsibility of the nursing staff is to obtain and administer your medications. They check behind the physician and pharmacist to ensure all medications are ordered appropriately.

Nurses will complete an assessment of you. The frequency of this depends on the nursing unit. This means asking you some routine questions like your name, birthday, what brought you into the hospital, etc. We will also ask you to do a few things (like squeeze our hands, wiggle your toes, etc.) and listen to your heart, lungs, and bowel sounds.

While doctors and their support staff round on you once a day, your nurse is there for you 24 hours per day. The medical team heavily relies on the nurse's ability to assess and monitor patients, and communicate concerns to them. We are responsible for alerting the physician with concerns related to your condition, lab values, medications, vital signs, etc.

We monitor you constantly throughout the day, but we also rely on you to tell us if you feel differently. Sudden unexpected pain, confusion, trouble breathing, numbness and tingling, weakness, or just something new are all things you want to tell your nurse.

Something else that the nurse is responsible for that takes up quite a bit of time is documentation. You may walk by the nurse's station and see all of the nurses at computers. I promise we don't check our email 100 times a day! Many hospitals have electronic charts, so basically everything we do is in a computer. From giving medications to reading patient notes to checking all of our orders, everything we do for you goes into your chart.

Nursing Interns and Students

During your stay, you may meet both nursing students and interns. Both nursing students and nursing interns are in nursing school and do not yet have their nursing licenses. They work with their clinical instructors and/or other nurses on the unit. Everything they do is checked and double-checked by others. They are in the process of learning how to be nurses. Nursing interns are typically between their junior and senior year of nursing school, working directly with one nurse from that particular unit.

Unlicensed Assistive Personnel

Whether they are trained as and called *certified nursing assistants* (CNAs) or *patient care technicians* (PCTs), to you as patient, they are one and the same. The people who hold these positions make up the unlicensed assistive staff who help out the nurses. They do not have a nursing license. While a nurse can do everything they can do, they cannot do all that a nurse does. This is why they may respond to a question or concern you have by saying, "I will let your nurse know." They are not trying to pass the buck by any means! There are just things that the nurse can address that they cannot.

Basically, their main focus is to help you with your *activities of daily living* (or ADLs as we call it in hospital lingo). They will help you with going to the bathroom, getting dressed for the day, walking around, bathing, eating, etc. They can also check your vital signs and your blood sugar. Depending on the hospital, some nursing assistants can do more than others. However, generally they are there to help you with your ADLs and to take your vital signs.

CNAs and PCTs are valuable members of the team. We all work together around the clock to make sure everyone's needs are met in a timely manner. Therefore, if the nurse and nursing assistant assigned to you are busy with two other patients and another nurse is available, he or she may come assist you so that you may go to the bathroom much faster than if they waited for the staff assigned to you.

Unit Secretaries

This staff member is at the nurse's station and answers phone calls, directs people who come up to the desk, page the medical team, stock cabinets, etc. This member of the health care team typically does not directly care for patients unless absolutely necessary.

Not all nursing units will have unit secretaries, thus leaving this task to the nurses and nursing assistants. Typically these members of the team are not staffed in the unit 24 hours a day, 7 days a week. Many times they are working when the unit is the busiest.

Nurses and Nursing FAQs

1. *I'm not comfortable with the nurse taking care of me during this shift. What do I do?*

The best way to address this is to ask to speak to the charge nurse first. If it is during normal business hours, you can always ask to speak to the nurse manager as well about your specific concerns. Typically, adjustments can be made but staffing does not always allow for this adjustment. Please don't suffer in silence—let someone know so the problem can be addressed. I discuss different ways to advocate for yourself in a later section.

2. *If I really liked my nurse or CNA/PCT from yesterday, can I request him or her again today?*

While we absolutely love it when patients request us by name, it cannot always be accommodated. Many times staffing allows us to grant these awesome requests, but just know that if there is someone who is really sick with something specific and your favorite nurse is the only one scheduled that day who is certified to deal with that particular equipment or need, they must be placed there. Otherwise, we love to make adjustments to make this work.

> **PATIENT TIP!** If you really want to say thank you, heartfelt cards really mean a lot to us. We keep them and look at them after a tough day to lift our spirits. Also, many hospitals have ways to recognize nurses with various awards and special recognitions.
>
> One example: the DAISY Award, for which patients and loved ones can nominate nurses. Feel free to ask or just pay attention as you or your loved one are going to the cafeteria, the waiting room, and so on, as nomination forms for these kinds of awards are usually in these areas. (See https://www. daisyfoundation.org/daisy-award)

3. *My nursing staff took amazing care of me and I want to get them something to thank them for this. What can I get them?*

Again, we love this! Just know that legally, we cannot accept anything of monetary value (like money or gift cards). However, we can accept food items (nurses love good food and coffee!), cards, flowers, and so on.

4. *My nurse said he or she "floated" to this unit. What does that mean?*

Nurses typically work on one unit, although depending on staffing you may have a nurse who has "floated" to your unit to care for patients. This means one unit was overstaffed and one was understaffed, so they are sharing the wealth by sending the nurse to the unit in need. While they may not typically care for patients on your unit, they are perfectly qualified to do so. Many hospitals have a "float pool," which is a group of nurses who do not have a home unit and go to where the need is every shift. So if a nurse says they are "floating to this unit," or they are a "float nurse," that's what it means.

5. *My nurse said he or she can't do something until he or she "has the order"—what does that mean?*

Legally, nurses cannot give medications, do any kind of therapy or procedure, feed you, get you out of bed, use various monitoring devices, or really do much of anything other than very basic things without an order from the physician. If you've ever heard a nurse say, "I'm just waiting for the doctor to put the order in," that is what this means. These orders are essential and are all located in your chart. They tell the entire nursing staff what they need to do or not do in specific circumstances as well as when they need to be notified.

> **PATIENT TIP!**   It is always okay to ask, "Who are you, again?" to someone who comes into your hospital room and starts asking questions. It is never rude; you need to know and fully understand your entire care team, especially if it is a new face.

Nurses and doctors work together as part of the health care team. We are constantly checking behind one another. Therefore, if a nurse notices that something is not ordered correctly or something is not right in your chart, they will alert the physician; the same is true with physicians alerting nurses. The lines of communication are always open and we are constantly working together to make sure everything in your chart is correct.

THE MEDICAL TEAM: DOCTORS AND OTHERS

There are many different kinds of doctors (more formally, *physicians*) and it can get pretty confusing. I'm going to outline various kinds of physicians and others on the medical team so that when someone comes into a room saying they are one of your doctors, you know exactly how they fit into your team.

Attending Physicians

These are the doctors who are running the show. They are in charge of your care overall, and will consult other doctors of other specialties as they see fit. Typically, they will see you every day, review your chart and plan of care, and touch base with the rest of the health care team.

Consulting Physicians

These are the other doctors that the attending doctor talks to (or "consults") for something specific outside of their realm. There is a process that the attending physician must follow to get doctors of a different practice outside their own to see you or your loved one. They speak directly with a physician of this group and explain the situation. This new "consulted physician" will closely look at the chart and come evaluate the patient personally.

Keep in mind: these are doctors who focus on specific body systems through their respective specialized practice. The cardiologist will deal with issues related to your heart, while the neurologist will deal with issue related to your brain, spinal cord, the rest of your nervous system, and (you might be surprised to learn) your muscles. If the neurologist comes into the room and you start asking them about the various blood pressure and other heart medicines, they may not answer and say it is up to the cardiologist.

The frequency at which you are seen by these specialists all depends on your location. If you are in a large hospital, you may be seen as often as daily. If you are in a smaller community hospital, these consulting physicians may only see you once.

In the tables on the following pages, I have listed most of specialties you are likely to encounter. There are two different subgroups of physicians (followed by more sub-subgroups!): medical specialties (listed on page 17) and surgical specialties (listed on page 20). A surgeon performs surgery, while a medical doctor does not. This distinction is very important. Many times doctors will talk about treating something medically versus surgically. Basically, *surgically* means that surgery will be performed and *medically* means that surgery will not be performed and the condition or issue will be managed with medicine and other therapies, not surgery. Some specialties allow physicians to care for patients in both a medical capacity and surgical capacity, but not all.

I have provided a list of most of the specialties of both surgical and medical doctors; however, you will note that some specialties could fit under both lists. Please keep that in mind when looking for which doctors are caring for you and/or your loved one! I recommend finding and highlighting the kind of physician(s) involved in your care.

Other Members of the Medical Team

These are some other members of the medical team that you may encounter during your stay.

Residents: These are medical doctors who are still going through their residency. They have completed four years of an undergraduate education and four years of medical school. Residents work within a team with an experienced physician in charge of them (called their "attending physician") and spend time in various specialties. Residencies can be as short as three years and as long as five years. They are physicians but are not out on their own yet. Typically only teaching hospitals have residents.

Medical Specialties and What the Specialists Do
NOTE: This is a general list and not all-encompassing

(Source: American Board of Medical Specialties, 2015)

A note about medical doctors

These physicians can work in both the hospital and in the clinic or outpatient setting. Because you or your loved one is in the hospital, you may see a physician who only works in the hospital. Therefore, if you need to continue seeing someone of this specialty after you are discharged (don't worry, they will tell you if you do!), you may see a different person.

Allergy and immunology: This group focuses on conditions or issues related to the immune system, which includes allergies. This can include things like immune responses to foods, to skin disorders like eczema, and even organ transplantation.

Anesthesiology: This group is most well known for being the doctors who manage sedation during surgery. They also specialize in pain management. If you're scheduled for surgery, typically one of these physicians will meet you beforehand and ask you very specific questions to make sure they have all of the information they need to safely sedate you for your operation. They also can be consulted to help out with patients who have pain that is very difficult to control. There are also highly trained and certified nurses, called CRNAs (certified registered nurse anesthetists), who work with anesthesiologists.

Dermatology: This group focuses on issues related to the skin, hair, and nails. They are more likely visited in an outpatient setting than in the hospital.

Emergency medicine: These are doctors who only work in the emergency department (ED). Emergency medicine encompasses so much and they see such a high volume of people that these physicians stay in the ED. When/If they decide the patient needs to stay in the hospital, they talk to another doctor who assumes care for the duration of the hospital stay. They know how to deal with very serious, life-threatening emergencies and work closely with support staff who are familiar with dealing with such. Some hospitals have separate EDs for the adult population, pediatric population, and even behavioral health population.

Family medicine: Occasionally these physicians work in the hospital, but many function in the clinic or outpatient setting. They can work with patients of all ages, whereas the internal medicine doctor only works with adults.

Hospitalists: These physicians solely work in the hospital, in most cases. Most are board-certified internists (see below). Their specialty is caring for patients in a hospital. Therefore, when you or your loved one is discharged, most likely you will not see this physician in the clinic or outpatient setting. They will assist in setting up follow-up appointments upon discharge with the appropriate physicians (for example, your primary care doctor or a specialist).

Internal medicine: An internal medicine doctor (or occasionally called an "internist") cares for a vast array of issues that can affect the adult patient. Just make sure you do not confuse them with an "intern"! Interns are further described later.

This medical specialty has 20 subspecialists as well as the general "internal medicine doctors." These subspecialties are adolescent medicine, adult congenital heart disease, advanced heart failure and transplant cardiology (heart transplants), cardiovascular disease (heart disease), clinical cardiac electrophysiology (issues with electrical issues involving the heart), critical care medicine (patients in the intensive care unit), endocrinology (diabetes and metabolism), gastroenterology (stomach, intestines, etc.), geriatric medicine (focuses on the elderly population), hematology (issues related to blood), hospice and palliative medicine (end of life and serious illnesses), infectious disease, interventional cardiology, medical oncology (cancer), nephrology (kidneys), pulmonary disease (lungs), rheumatology (joint disorders), sleep medicine, sports medicine, and transplant hematology (liver transplants).

Neurology: This group works with patients who are suffering from a disease of the nervous system. This includes both the spinal cord and the brain. They treat patients who have had various kinds of strokes, suffer from seizures, neurodevelopmental disabilities, and even brain injuries. They can specialize in child neurology as well.

Pathology: This group looks at and interprets disease in your tissues or bodily fluids. If you've ever heard someone say, "We need to check the pathology first," or "We have to wait for pathology to get back before we know what to do," they are talking about sending the sample to these doctors. They take a look at whatever it may be (anything from a piece of someone's brain to a lesion on someone's pinky toe) and classify it. They communicate and collaborate with the rest of the medical team to determine the best course of action.

Pediatrics: This group will care for patients under the age of 18. These patients will typically be on a pediatric unit ("the peds floor") or a pediatric intensive care unit (the "PICU") with specialized nursing care, as it is a specialized patient population. There are 19 total subspecialties of pediatric physician, many of which are the same as the internal medicine specialty listed above. Additional subspecialties for pediatrics include child abuse pediatrics, developmental behavioral pediatrics, medical toxicology, and neonatal–perinatal medicine.

Physical medicine and rehabilitation: This group's focus is to optimize function for patients whose functional capabilities have been compromised for various reasons and has various subspecialties (for example, spinal cord medicine, pain medicine, and brain injury medicine). You may hear this doctor referred to as "the rehab doctor."

Psychiatry and mental health: This group deals with the diagnosis and treatment of a vast array of mental illnesses. There are quite a few subspecialties, including addiction psychiatry, child and adolescent psychiatry, and even forensic psychiatry.

Radiology: This group specializes in interpreting various images or scans. If you've ever heard someone say "We need to wait until the radiologist takes a look at it," that means they need to wait for someone from this group to look at the scan and interpret exactly what is going on. Not only do they interpret, they also can make recommendations and suggest treatments as well. These scans are so complex that there must be an entire specialty devoted to interpreting them.

Surgical Specialties and What the Surgeons Do

NOTE: This is a general list and not all-encompassing

(Source: American College of Surgeons website, accessed Nov. 19, 2015)

A note about surgeons

Surgeons are responsible for the care of patients receiving the surgery. They perform this care in three phases: before surgery, during surgery, and after surgery. Many times additional physicians from another specialties are also caring for the same patient, but the surgeon will focus on the aspects of care directly related to the surgery in which they performed. In addition to surgery in the operating room, they can also perform various procedures in their office locations and on nursing units with appropriate equipment and support. While many medical doctors only work inpatient (meaning they only see patients in the hospital), most surgeons will prepare you for surgery before admission, perform the surgery, and care for you after the surgery, even well after your hospitalization is complete. You will most likely see them in their office as well as in the hospital.

Typically, surgeons belong to one of the following specialties. They can further specialize in a sub-specialty as well. For example, someone can be a neurosurgeon with a specific sub-specialization in operating on brain tumors. Please note that I have not listed all subspecialties; this is a general list.

General surgeon: This surgeon performs a broad range of various surgeries that involve, but are not limited to, surgeries of the soft tissues, skin, gastrointestinal system, vascular system, head, neck, breast, and the endocrine system.

Thoracic surgeon: This surgeon works in the thoracic (or chest) region. They specifically perform surgery on tumors on the esophagus, chest wall, and lungs, as well as surgery related to coronary artery disease. This can include coronary artery bypass graft surgery or heart valve replacement/repair surgery.

Colon and rectal surgeon: This surgeon focuses on treating various problems in the colon, rectum, anal canal, and perianal area both medically and surgically.

Neurological surgeon (or neurosurgeon): This group focuses on your nervous system. They can operate on your brain, spinal cord, and the vascular structures that support them.

Obstetrics and gynecological surgery: Not only does this group care for pregnant patients, they are also trained to deliver babies. They are also able to surgically and medically treat issues that affect the female reproductive system.

Ophthalmic surgeon: This surgeon works on the eyes and vision; in fact, these surgeons are the only ones who can diagnose and treat all eye and vision problems! They can provide vision services, but they also perform surgery and various treatments. They are different from optometrists in that they can perform surgery and have a medical degree.

Oral and maxillofacial surgeon: This surgeon focuses on the face and jaw (which is what the maxillo part means) regions. They treat a wide variety of issues affecting this area of your body, including injuries, cancers, cysts, and defects, and they can even take out wisdom teeth and put in dental implants.

Orthopedic surgeons: These surgeons focus on the musculoskeletal system. It's a pretty large system, so there are many subspecialties that range across hands, trauma, foot and ankle, and joint replacement. These surgeries can be because of birth defects, accidents, infections, tumors, or degenerative conditions, just to name a few reasons.

Otolaryngology surgeon: This surgeon works in your ears. He or she can provide both medical and surgical treatment to the ear and connecting structures.

Pediatric surgeon: This doctor works with children (people under 18) needing surgery. Because kids are continually growing, they need to have a specialized surgeon to meet their needs. Pediatric surgeons can further specialize in neonates (infants or even premature babies), oncology, trauma, and even prenatal care.

Plastic surgeon: These surgeons do much more than cosmetic surgery. They can manage complex wounds, perform skin grafts, and transplant tissue.

Urologist: This doctor takes care of issues related to the genitourinary (organs related to the genitals and urinary system and adrenal glands) both medically and surgically.

Vascular surgeon: This surgeon deals with problems that affect the arteries and veins that course through your entire body.

Interns: An intern is someone currently in the first year of their residency.

> **PATIENT TIP!**   Do not confuse interns with internists or internal medicine doctors!

Medical students: A medical student is someone who has completed four years of undergraduate education and is in the four years of medical school. They are not yet physicians and are typically working with a resident and/or attending physician.

Physician's assistants (PAs) and nurse practitioners (NPs): Other absolutely essential members of the health care team are PAs and NPs. Many work with a specific physician or group of physicians. They see patients, write orders, prescribe medications, work on your care plans, and consult with the rest of the health care team. PAs and NPs can work in the hospital, clinics, and offices.

> **PATIENT TIP!**   These providers are typically referred to as an "NP" or a "PA".

More about Doctors

How Doctors Schedule Work

Most doctors work Monday through Friday from 8:00 a.m. to 5:00 p.m., both in and out of the hospital. For the hours outside of this, doctors within a practice take turns being on-call. So if you need something at midnight one night, your nurse will call the doctor on-call, and if the doctor is not your doctor, he or she is typically a partner of your doctor. Nurses call the doctor on-call for various reasons, such as to obtain an order for a medication, to ask a clarifying question, to update them on a change that has occurred, and so forth. When your doctor is back the next morning, the doctor on-call will update your doctor about what happened overnight. This is common practice because it is not feasible for one doctor to be available 24 hours a day, 7 days a week. This allows the team to have time off and rest.

Doctors round on their patients once per day. Some physicians start rounding very early in the morning so they can be done sooner in the evening. This depends on the facility, but you should expect to see your physician once per day.

When Doctors See You

Doctors round on their patients whenever it fits into their schedule. Their schedules are typically unpredictable and can change at a moment's notice. Your doctor may be responsible for responding to codes (when someone's heart stops or they stop breathing) in the hospital, which would change what time they could come and see you. Emergencies and urgent situations occur, which makes it very hard to predict when they will be coming by.

The order in which physicians choose to see their patients is up to them. In my experience, I have noted that many physicians like to round first on the sickest patients or ones who are actively having problems that need to be urgently addressed.

If you've had surgery, after the surgery, while you're still waking up in the recovery unit, the surgeon typically goes and chats with your family member. Depending on the severity of the surgery and how you did, you may not see them again until they round the next day.

> **Rounding/Rounds:** When a member of your health care team comes to see you while you are in the hospital. Most team members, except for the nurse, will round once per day. They will review your chart and care plan, make adjustments as needed, and speak with you directly. The nurse and members of the nursing staff will round many times each day.

Physician FAQs

1. *What does it mean when a doctor says they've "signed off"?*

   When a doctor "signs off" on a patient, that means they are a consulting physician and have provided whatever service addressed the patient's need, and it is no longer necessary for them to continue seeing that patient. While they are still available for questions, they will no longer round every day on you.

2. *Can't my primary care doctor just come see me in the hospital while I'm here instead of these new doctors?*

   In some rare instances, this does occur. However, for a physician to work in a particular facility (meaning have access to all private medical information, access to the building, ability place orders, etc.) he or she must have "privileges" there. He or she must go through the security clearance process that all employees go through, plus multiple other steps, to be able to have privileges. In saying that, most physicians who have an outpatient practice focusing on internal medicine or family practice typically only practice there and not in the hospital as well. Therefore, it is not as easy as he or she just walking into the building to care for you. There is a lot of behind-the-scenes work and clearance that must be done first and typically cannot be done on a case-by-case basis.

3. *Who updates my primary care doctor, telling him or her that I'm in the hospital and about my stay?*

This is another thing that can vary from facility to facility, but you can ask your nurse to call your doctor's office to leave a message for them, alerting him or her that you have been hospitalized. Many times, after a hospitalization, the physician will want you to follow up with your primary doctor afterward.

4. *My doctor came to see me and I forgot my questions I wanted to ask him/her. Can they come back to see me?*

While occasionally they can make time to come back, this is not always feasible. Physicians and their team typically have a long list of patients to see throughout their day, or they may have left the hospital to go to their outpatient office, if they have one. If this does happen, the quickest way to get in touch with them is to have the nurse page the physician, then have you or your loved one speak with them on the phone. While it would be great if they were on the unit at all times, sitting at a desk, this is rarely the case. They are typically walking around the hospital, rounding on other patients, in a procedure, or at another facility.

There are many other members of the health care team in addition to the nurses and doctors. I will outline a few different kinds of therapists and their role within the team. While every patient will have a nurse and doctor taking care of them, not everyone on this list will see every patient.

Physical Therapists

Many patients in the hospital are seen by a physical therapist. This person typically holds a doctorate degree in physical therapy (DPT), although some have a master's degree, and a few have their bachelor's degree. They go through a grueling course load and must pass certification exams to become a licensed physical therapist.

Not every patient will be seen by a physical therapist, but most will. If you've had surgery, undergone a major illness, have been in bed quite a bit, etc., the doctor will usually order the physical therapist to come see you and check you out. The reason they have to come see you initially (even if you're doing great!) is that many insurance companies and Medicare/Medicaid require them to evaluate you if you have been through certain procedures or diagnoses, and rely on their recommendations for your plan of care and safe return home.

The goal of the physical therapist is to improve your movement, mobility, and function. The therapist wants to make sure it is safe for you to go home. Typically, he or she will ask you about things like where you live, if you have stairs, if you have support systems in place, etc. If you were completely independent and pain-free with movement before your admission, the goal is to get you back to functional status.

They first assess you and see what your needs are, develop a treatment plan and frequency for it, and go from there. Depending on your needs, you may not be seen by PT (hospital lingo for physical therapy) every day. PT may see you every other day, twice a week, etc. Also, it may not be the same person every day. He or she can give you exercises to do on your own and also let the nursing staff know the best and safest way to get you up and moving around.

If you or your loved one is bedbound, physical therapy can still work for you! Physical therapy even goes to the neonatal intensive care unit and works with the tiny babies! It's truly amazing. So, if you're confined to the bed, they will still come and see what all you can and cannot do and develop a treatment plan based on your specific needs.

Occupational Therapists

While physical therapy works to get your movement and mobility maximized, occupational therapy (OT) focuses on getting you back to your baseline with your activities of daily living (your ADLs). This means feeding yourself, going to the bathroom, cleaning yourself, etc. This can be much more complicated and complex than people realize, which is why OT is so necessary.

Most occupational therapists hold a doctorate or master's degree. They also must get through a tough course load and pass an exam to be licensed.

Again, OT will only see you if the doctor orders it. Many times this is necessary and appropriate, but again, not every single patient will see them. They have a similar routine as the physical therapy team. They'll assess you, develop a treatment plan and frequency, and get to work! They may help you eat, bathe, or walk. If working with therapy really tires you out, they may coordinate their time with the physical therapy team so they both can see you at the same time so it does not overwhelm you.

Speech Therapists

Speech therapists (STs) are another member of our health care team. They focus on issues with swallowing and communication. Like the rest of your health care squad, speech therapists are also highly educated. Speech therapists must have their master's degree and also have to pass a strenuous licensing exam to practice.

This is another member of the health care team who does not necessarily see every patient in the hospital. It is up to the physician to consult the speech therapist as they see fit. Many times the speech therapist will evaluate you or your loved one for impaired swallowing initially. (Speech therapists deal with swallowing issues? Yes! Take a look at the box on pages 30–31 about safe swallowing and nutrition.) This therapist will develop a treatment plan, determine the frequency of seeing you, and continue to follow you throughout your stay. However, if you also have impaired communication skills because of your reason for admission (again, strokes are a good example of this), they will also cognitively evaluate you and work on communication skills as well.

Another member of the team is called the respiratory therapist. They work closely with the nursing staff and physicians to determine the best course of treatment for you from a cardiopulmonary standpoint. They take care of patients of all ages, from the premature babies in the neonatal intensive care unit to the elderly. They work in many different units all across the hospital and some even work in the outpatient setting as well.

Respiratory therapists know all of the ins and outs of oxygen therapy, which is very complex. They are very knowledgeable about breathing machines (also called ventilators), different ways to deliver oxygen therapy, and many medications for your heart and lungs. Not every patient will require a visit from this member of the team, but many will.

OTHER MEMBERS OF THE HEALTH CARE TEAM

Pharmacists

This is one member of the team who is working hard behind the scenes, but you may never actually see them. Most hospitals have a pharmacy within their walls, and within this pharmacy are pharmacists and pharmacy technicians.

This person is another doctorate-prepared member of the team. They must go through an extremely rigorous process to become a pharmacist and many complete residency programs for additional training. Pharmacists can also specialize in various fields (like oncology).

Speech Therapy Is Not Just about Speaking: When Safe Swallowing Is Impaired

From strokes to trauma to being on a breathing machine (or ventilator), your ability to safely swallow can easily be compromised. Many people believe that if food or fluids are "going down the wrong pipe," the cough reflex will kick in and you'll know if you're choking. However, that is not the case. Sometimes food or liquid can slip down into your trachea (or "windpipe") without you even knowing it. This is called "silent aspiration" and it can be very dangerous. Depending on what caused the impaired swallowing in the first place (a stroke, for example) that cough reflex can be suppressed and you can get food and/or fluid in your lungs without having a clue. This can lead to pneumonia, which is a serious complication. This is why it is essential that a thorough evaluation by a highly educated individual be completed before you or your loved one eats or drinks anything if your health care team is concerned about swallowing. It is a matter of safety.

Many family members and loved ones become very concerned if the patient has not eaten anything for days. While some patients can say they are hungry, many are not thinking about food at all.

Think about when you're sick and feel terrible. Are you usually craving a meal? Many times when something traumatic or major occurs in the body, eating is not always the body's top priority. Seeing a loved one go a few days without eating can be more stressful for the person watching than the person who is lying in the bed. While proper nutrition is essential to healing, it is absolutely necessary to ensure that the patient can safely swallow food first. It does no good, and actually does serious harm, if it goes down the trachea instead of the esophagus.

Different ways to get nutrition

The best situation is when patients are able to eat regular food and drink regular liquids. Oral is always the preferred route for medications, so we want people to be able to eat and drink as soon as possible! If the patient cannot safely swallow normal thin liquids and normal foods, the next step would be a modified diet. In this situation, the food can be a mechanical soft texture or pureed texture, and the liquids can be thickened to a honey or nectar thickness to aid in safe swallowing. However, despite modifications there are still situations in which it is not safe to eat or drink. In these situations, the health care team may recommend enteral nutrition, also known as tube feedings.

Enteral nutrition (tube feeding)

Enteral nutrition is administered through this tube to safely supply food and water past the vocal cords and directly to the stomach or beginning of the small intestines. A nurse inserts this tube and this tube can stay in for a long period of time. It sounds aggressive, but it is actually the least aggressive option at this point. Typically, the speech therapist continues to work with the patient with the goal that the tube will eventually be removed and regular food (modified or not) can be resumed.

However, there are times in which the medical team and speech therapy team believe that either normal swallowing will never resume or it will be an extended period of time in which this will occur. In these instances, a tube can be surgically inserted into the abdomen to administer the same feeding directly into the stomach. This is called a **p**ercutaneous **e**ndoscopic **g**astrostomy tube (or *PEG tube* for short). This is done because after a certain amount of time, the tube that goes through the nose can cause irritation to the tissues of the nose and throat.

Parenteral nutrition (TPN)

In cases in which the stomach or gastrointestinal tract cannot tolerate food or liquids, it can be administered intravenously (in your veins). This is called parenteral nutrition. However, this is definitely the last option and never preferred. It is hard on your vein and is nothing like normal nutrition that is absorbed through the gut. Many people believe it's just the same thing as food but in IV form, but it is not. Tube feeding and regular food are highly preferred to this route.

If you or your loved one is on parenteral nutrition, I don't want you to think it is unsafe. It is safe. However, your health care team (especially your speech therapist and registered dietician) will be constantly looking to wean off of that and on to enteral or oral nutrition as soon as possible because it is highly superior and provides much better outcomes.

A pharmacist reviews every medication that is prescribed for you and every other patient in the hospital. Not everyone sees a speech therapist, but a pharmacist lays eyes on every single patient's chart multiple times. They make sure the medication, and all of its ingredients, are safe for you to receive. They compare your medications and their ingredients to your list of allergies (including food allergies and interactions), all other medications you're receiving, and they even check your lab values to make sure your kidneys, liver, etc. can appropriately process the medication.

A physician orders a medication, the pharmacist reviews it then signs off on it, and then finally the nurse can administer it. If the pharmacist finds that the medication interacts with another medication you're receiving or if they find that, for whatever reason, the medication is not safe for you to receive, they will speak with the physician personally and figure out another option.

Pharmacists are highly educated and an essential part of the team. While patients don't interact with them frequently, your health care team members speak with them many times throughout the day to make sure you're getting the best and safest medication possible.

Registered Dieticians

A registered dietician is someone who is there to optimize your nutritional status. This person has either a bachelor's or master's degree, has completed many clinical hours, and has passed a licensing exam.

Dieticians see people from the premature baby to the adolescent on the pediatric floor with an eating disorder to the elderly man in the intensive care unit who just had a massive stroke. They work closely with the speech therapy team and the food service team to ensure that you or your loved one is getting the proper nutrition of the proper consistency.

As previously discussed, some patients in the hospital are unable to swallow regular food. This can be because of many conditions, like throat or neck surgery, stroke, being on a ventilator or trauma, to name a few. In these situations, the physician will order enteral nutrition or tube feeding. When a physician orders this, the registered dietician (or RD) will look at the patient's chart closely and determine which formula will best meet their needs. They look at lab values, medications, diagnoses, intake and output, and other factors., to determine this. They reevaluate this frequently and change the formula as needed.

They also work closely with patients who have specific dietary needs. They work with patients with kidney failure, patients with uncontrolled diabetes, on chemotherapy, or patients who are just not getting their nutritional requirements. They work with the nursing staff and the food service team to determine the best foods and supplements to improve nutrition.

Chaplains

The chaplains who work in the hospital are different than chaplains at the church down the street. Typically, to be a hospital chaplain you must have a bachelor's degree in a field like counseling or theology. However, many hospitals require their chaplains to have a Masters of Divinity and be credentialed through an accrediting body.

Hospital chaplains do quite a few things. They can lead services at the hospital chapel. Many are notaries and will assist patients and their loved ones in creating and signing a health care power of attorney document (if the patient is of sound mind). They also provide spiritual support to patients, visitors, and even staff members. Typically, they respond to emergencies or when patients and loved ones receive particularly bad news. Many round on nursing units to see which patients could use some spiritual support. They also can help patients and families mentally and emotionally process all that is going on while they're in the hospital, as it can be pretty overwhelming.

Something else the chaplains are great at doing is getting the right spiritual support person in the room. While they are there to support anyone of any religion, some people prefer someone from their particular religion. The people who work in the chaplaincy office know how to get a hold of religious officials from outside the hospital. Depending on your location, they can try to find local rabbis, pastors, priests, Buddhist monks, or call a local mosque for you or your loved one. Your spiritual health and support is essential, and they help the health care team facilitate it successfully.

Licensed Social Workers

Social workers are another essential member of the health care team. While they can be bachelor's prepared, many have their master's degree as well. They must also pass a licensing exam to practice.

Social workers focus on helping you or your loved ones get back to life from a practical standpoint after leaving the hospital. They help you figure out your finances and help with family issues, including coping and support. While not every single patient sees or needs a social worker, they work closely with the nursing staff to identify the patients who may need to see them. They want to make sure going home is safe and realistic. This means that they can provide resources and options for people dealing with abuse, coping with various illnesses, or having various financial concerns, just to name a few. They are an invaluable resource to all patients.

Case Managers, Care Coordinators

While case managers work closely with social workers, they have a different function. To be a certified case manager, a bachelor's degree must be held. (Many case managers who work in hospitals are actually nurses!) Case managers focus on care coordination from a big picture point of view. So, nurses coordinate care within the health care team at the hospital during this particular admission, and case managers coordinate care within the patient's entire experience. They work closely with Medicare, Medicaid, insurance companies, nursing homes, rehab facilities, skilled care facilities, etc. They facilitate the transfer from the hospital to wherever home may be. If you or your loved one needs to be transferred to another hospital or nursing home, they facilitate this as well.

In short, case managers manage care resources. They identify what kind of support services you or your loved one will need upon discharge and facilitate the process. They work closely with the health care team to identify these needs as early as possible. They might talk to the physical therapist about their recommendations for the patient's discharge. They want to know if the patient will be able to go to a rehab facility or if the physical therapist is recommending a nursing home, rehab, home health, or specific medical equipment for the home upon discharge. Along with the rest of the team, they will communicate these things to you or your loved one and get the paperwork and everything started early so that the discharge process is as smooth as it can be.

As you can tell, your health care team is comprised of many highly educated and licensed individuals. While they all have different functions and specialties, they all work together to make sure that you or your loved one is getting the specialized support that you require for success.

Speaking of you and your loved one….

Families, Loved Ones, and Visitors

Some of the most important members of your health care team are the people who make up your support system It is essential to your healing to have emotional support from others. We always want your support system, however you define it, to be with you as much as possible as you heal.

We also realize that having visitors can make it difficult to rest. Please let the nursing staff know if you'd like us to limit visitors. We will gladly tell you visitors to come back at another time. You are the priority. Your rest, your health, and your healing come above all things—including entertaining guests, no matter how close they are to you. Please rest assured that your nursing staff is very comfortable and used to kindly asking people to leave so you can rest. Just give us the green light and we will very kindly and graciously ask people to step out.

Additionally, if there are people who you do not want to visit you, please let the staff know. Word can travel fast between family, friends, work, or prayer circles at church and people can show up that you did not anticipate. While it may be with good intention that people want to visit, they may not realize how cumbersome it can be with many visitors. Please let your nurse know. We can always put a sign on the door or leave a message with the medical unit receptionist that there are visitor limitations at this time. Again, your health is the priority.

As you can tell, there are a lot of people who make up your health care team, all with very specific roles. Regardless of each person's role, you and your needs are at the center of it all. Because there are so many different people on the team, communication is essential. Therefore, if you do not understand something or someone's role, please speak up and ask. You will not offend anyone. We understand that you see a lot of new faces all the time!

SECTION 2

YOUR HOSPITAL STAY: GETTING ADMITTED, TREATED, AND DISCHARGED

Now that you know at least something about all of the members of the health care team, let's walk though and talk about the actual hospital and the main ways you'll get to be what we call an "inpatient."

Here's what you can learn about in this section:

▸ Your four most likely routes for your hospital admission: the emergency department, after surgery, through a doctor's office, or through a procedural area.

▸ The many parts and departments of the typical hospital.

▸ Some essential (need-to-know!) topics: equipment you're likely to encounter; hospital food; and in-hospital medication issues, including details about their administration and their timing and critical information on pain meds.

▸ Three basic processes that come into play while you're there, while you move around, and while you're leaving: communication, transfers, and discharges.

You may notice that people do not call it the "emergency room" anymore. The official title is the "emergency department," as it is an entire department and not one room. It is frequently called the "ED."

The staff in the ED will look at each patient who comes through the doors and decide based on the situation how quickly the patient will be seen by a physician. This is called "triage." Basically, the more emergent and serious the situation, the faster the patient is seen. Ideally, the ED is only used for true emergencies.

The staff in the ED is working as fast as possible to see all of the patients and treat them in the appropriate order. While you may be in one room for getting a large cut on your arm and require stitches, the person in the room next to you may be having a heart attack. Therefore, the nurses and doctors will attend to the guy next door first and once he is stabilized, they will attend to your arm. Coming to this department for treatment is all about treating the sickest or most injured patients first.

PATIENT TIP!   While we hate to wait in most other situations, waiting in the ED is a good thing. This means you are not the sickest person in the department. Because people come into the department at unpredictable times, you may wait a long time during one visit and a short time during another visit. The ED does not function like an outpatient clinic with appointments. Please, expect to wait unless you really are experiencing a serious emergency.

---

1. *Who is my doctor at this time?*

   If you're in the ED, the ED physician at that time is your only doctor. The ED physician determines if you need to stay in the hospital, and if so they call another doctor to admit you and assume your care. They care for patients in terms of hours, not days, and are focused on treating patients in emergent situations as well as determining which patients need continued monitoring and treatment, and which can go home.

   Which doctor this ED physician calls to assume your care varies based upon your condition. While this varies, many times an internal medicine doctor will be in charge. The doctor who takes over your care, regardless of specialty, is called your attending physician.

2. *What happens after they decide I need to get admitted?*

   After the ED doctor decides you need to be in the hospital and calls another physician who will take over your care, that physician requests a bed in the unit he or she would like you to be on. Occasionally, you may need to wait for a bed to become available.

   The unit that will be receiving you prepares for your arrival. They make sure the room is ready and decide which nurse will be your primary nurse. The nurse caring for you in the ED will communicate with your new nurse about what brought you into the hospital, what they did for you in the ED, and the current plan of care. You will then be brought to your new room.

After Surgery

Another way you can end up in a hospital bed is by staying overnight (or longer) after surgery. Your doctor will decide if you need to stay in the hospital after your surgery and typically you are well aware of this prior to going to the operating room.

Patients typically come in at their scheduled time, go to the pre-operative admission unit, then to the operating room, then to the recovery room, and then finally up to their hospital room. This typically means a day full of "hurry up and wait" for your loved ones!

In most cases, your surgeon is going to be your attending physician. A typical example of this situation is if you are being admitted for a particular surgery, like a heart surgery. The surgeon will typically be your attending physician in this case. In less common situations, a different physician is your attending physician.

Through a Doctor's Office

Sometimes people become patients in the hospital because their outpatient doctor felt it was necessary to bypass the emergency department and go straight to a hospital room. Your doctor calls the hospital and secures a bed for you and you come straight up to a room. This is the least common way to become a patient in a hospital, but it does occasionally occur.

Through a Procedural Area

Another way you may become a patient in a hospital is after a procedure. There are quite a few different procedural areas in various facilities. These can include the catheter ("cath") lab, interventional radiology, and dialysis units, to name a few. Your health care team may decide you need to stay in the hospital for a certain period of time after going through a specific procedure (a heart catheterization, for example) before going home.

Inter-Facility Transfer

Hospitals can be very different. Some are very large and have many different units and departments, while others are very small with fewer resources. Smaller hospitals are not always able to take care of everything that may happen. If you go to the nearest hospital when an emergency occurs and they discover that you need equipment or services that

---

Patient Classifications

There are terms for when someone is receiving care from a health care team in various settings. Please see below for the three patient classifications!

Inpatient: A patient who stays in the hospital while being treated; where the patient stays while being treated in the hospital.

Observation status: When your health care team is deciding if your needs can be addressed by being admitted as an inpatient or as an outpatient. This can mean you'll be in the hospital for up to 24 hours while this decision is being made.

Outpatient: Place where a patient receives care in a given setting; a patient who gets care in a given setting: a clinic, procedural area, same-day surgery center, and so on. You go home once care is given: there are no overnight stays in an outpatient facility!

---

they do not have (for example, a cardiac catheterization for a heart attack at a hospital without a cath lab or a brain surgery for a tumor removal at a hospital without a neurosurgeon), they will transfer you to the nearest facility with what you need. Doctors working with the rest of the health care team at both the current facility and the one you will go to will get together and get you to where you need to be as fast as possible. Typically, you will bypass the emergency department and go straight to a hospital room, provided it is available. Depending on the situation, you may go from one facility to another in an ambulance.

A similar process occurs if you or a loved one is a patient in a rehab facility, long-term care facility, or skilled nursing facility. The staff at both the current facility and receiving facility will discuss the best way to get you where you need to go.

THE PARTS AND DEPARTMENTS OF A HOSPITAL

Of the many different parts and departments in a hospital, here are those that you are most likely to encounter or at least hear about.

The Emergency Department (ED)

This is where you go for emergencies when you are outside of the hospital. You are either sent home or admitted to the hospital, as we previously discussed.

Levels of Care

There are three levels of care in the hospital: intensive care, step-down (or intermediate), and the regular nursing floor. Intensive care requires the closest monitoring of the most unstable patients. It is considered the highest level of care because the monitoring is constant and patients can be very unstable. If you or a loved one requires a higher level of care, that means the nurse needs to be available to watch you or your loved one more closely.

The Regular Nursing Floor

Typically called "the floor," this is where most hospital patients will reside. The general hospital floor is called the "med–surg floor," meaning patients with both medical and surgical issues will receive their care here. Patients are not critically ill, but are not well enough to be at home.

There are various nursing floors that specialize in certain areas. For example, many hospitals have a cardiology floor, oncology floor, neurology floor, renal floor, etc. These are wonderful because the nurses on these floors are very familiar with a specific patient population. For example, if you came into the ED with a heart attack, typically you are sent to the cardiology floor afterwards. These nurses take care of patients with heart conditions all day every day, and are very familiar with this patient population and their needs.

When you are admitted to the hospital, the doctor along with the nursing staff seek to put you on an appropriate unit that best suits your needs. Maybe the renal unit just got renovated and has really nice big rooms, but if you had a stroke you will want to be on the stroke unit! Those nurses work closely with neurologists and neurosurgeons all the time and are very familiar with the potential complications of stroke patients. Not to say that the renal nurses cannot take care of stroke patients, but it is preferred that nurses who are familiar with a specific patient population do so on a regular basis. This allows nurses to provide customized expert care.

Because patients on these units are considered the most stable, the nurses caring for these patients will have the highest nurse-to-patient ratio. Meaning, your nurse can be caring for you and as many as seven other people at the same time. If closer monitoring is required, the patient will need to be moved to a higher level of care. This means they need to be transferred to one of the following two units.

Step-Down Unit or Intermediate Unit

Patients on this unit are not quite critically ill, but need closer monitoring than can be provided on a medical–surgical unit. Step-down units can be specialized (pulmonary, cardiac, or neurological are common); however, not all hospitals have these units. Nurses on these units have a lower nurse-to-patient ratio than the floor nurses, but not as low as the critical care nurses. Most stepdown units will continuously monitor their patients on various machines like a heart monitor, pulse oximetry monitor, and frequent blood pressure assessments.

Critical Care, Intensive Care, or ICU (Intensive Care Unit)

Whatever it is called in a given hospital, this unit is for the very sick patients. The closest monitoring is done here; physicians are typically on this unit 24 hours a day. Typically one nurse is assigned for every one to two patients. However some patients are so unstable that they require a nurse dedicated only to them. Patients are frequently on various drips to keep their vital signs stable, have various tubes or drains to manage frequently, and/or are on a breathing tube to help them breathe. The nurse, along with the rest of the health care team, is responsible for managing all of these things.

The goal is to get you out of this unit as quickly as possible and only admit you here if it's absolutely necessary. There are a lot of monitors, tubes, and wires, all which can cause confusion or delirium. The faster you get out of the ICU, the better!

These units can also be specialized, depending on the size of the hospital. There are medical, surgical, trauma, neuroscience, cardiac, and transplant intensive care units to name a few. The specialization is wonderful because the staff on the units can focus on the specific needs of the patients.

Pre-Operative (Pre-Op)

Pre-op is where you go before surgery. They give you the medicine they want you to have before surgery (like antibiotics), put in IVs and other lines, and do all of the very necessary last minute things to get you ready for the operating room. Some facilities allow family to be in the pre-operative area.

Operating Room (OR)

This is where surgery happens. There are many people in the OR helping with each case. The surgeon is in charge, who may have a physician's assistant or nurse practitioner assisting them, an anesthesiologist or CRNA (a highly skilled and trained nurse with an advanced degree who provides anesthesia care during some surgeries), as well as scrub technicians, and a nurse or two, depending on what is going on.

Depending on the surgery, there may be more than one surgeon and additional support staff involved. Typically, patients are given meds in the pre-op phase that will relax them, then once they are in the OR and everyone is ready to go, they are sedated. During surgery, family/loved ones are invited to the waiting room and updated periodically throughout the case.

Recovery Room or PACU (Post-Anesthesia Recovery Unit)

After surgery is done and the health care team starts waking you back up, they immediately take you to the recovery unit. These nurses make sure you come out of anesthesia properly and control your pain. Depending on the length and type of surgery, you can be in the recovery unit for a very short period of time or a few hours. Once you have woken up, you will be taken to your hospital room or sent home, if appropriate. Loved ones and family members typically are not permitted in the PACU. This is an open unit, full of other patients recovering from their surgeries. Therefore, most facilities will have the family wait in the waiting room until the patient is either up in their hospital room or getting cleared to go home.

Procedural Areas

Hospitals contain other units in which procedures take place. This can include endoscopy, the catheter ("cath") lab, or an area dedicated to "special procedures." Patients usually come to these units for their procedure, then to the recovery room, and finally back to their hospital room or home if appropriate.

Other Areas for Tests and Scans

Patients can visit various other departments for tests or scans as well. This can include the radiology department, nuclear medicine, or the MRI department to name a few. This is another area where patients come for their scheduled test or scan, and then leave for their room or home, if appropriate.

SOME ASSORTED IN-HOSPITAL ESSENTIALS ALL PATIENTS NEED TO KNOW

Equipment Most Likely to Encounter

When you're in the hospital, many patients have multiple lines and tubes attached. Here are a few short explanations of some of the things we use on a regular basis.

Every hospital room should have a call bell that is within arm's reach so if you need to speak with a staff member you are able to do so quickly. However, if you have activated your call bell to request the nurse or nurse's aide and no one has come to your room within a maximum 20 minutes, please use the call bell again. While every single patient is important to us, the message that you needed something may not have been relayed, or an emergency occurred and it had to be addressed first. Do not feel like you're bothering the staff by doing this. It is important to us that your needs are met.

Additionally, if you or your loved one does not have the strength or dexterity to physically push the call bell, please let the staff know. Most units have adaptive devices that will enable you to alert the staff when you have needs.

The IV Pump

This device is used to give you a certain amount of a liquid medication straight into your vein over a certain period of time. You can get fluids, antibiotics, and many other things with the help of this machine. It is attached to a rolling pole and can go with you wherever you may go (except in the shower or on the stairs!).

One of the functions of an IV pump is to alert the nursing staff when it has run out of medication, is unable to deliver the medication (for example, if there is a kink in the line), or if the battery is dying. If your pump starts to beep, please press your call bell. Nurses can't always hear that beep, especially if your door is closed and the TV is on. These pumps are not connected to anything at the nurse's station to alert us. We hear what you hear, but we are typically walking around the entire unit so it is not nearly as loud (or annoying!) to us. If someone has not come to address the pump in a timely fashion, please put your call light on to alert your nurse.

Also, do not, under any circumstances, touch the buttons on the IV pump. You can accidently give yourself too much or not enough of a medication. Depending on the medication, this can cause serious effects or problems. Please use your call bell to alert the staff that it is beeping.

If you see that the IV or its tubing is dislodged or that the sheets are wet with liquid, hear the pump beeping, or feel pain and soreness around the area where the IV is going into your arm, please immediately notify the nurse. Never try to reconnect something that appears to be dislodged. Most of the tubing looks very similar and we wouldn't want you to accidentally connect one kind of tubing to a totally different kind! Just because something looks like it connects does not mean it does, and just because two things fit together does not mean they should!

I will tell you the age-old example of why this can be a really big problem. This example is told to health care professionals across the country during hospital orientation to make sure they educate their patient's support system appropriately:

A patient was receiving oxygen in his nose in a tube that looks similar to the tubing that connects the IV to his arm (clear tubing with a circumference slightly smaller than a drinking straw). Somehow, both the IV tubing and the oxygen tubing became dislodged. Not wanting to bother the nurse, a family member just "reconnected everything." However, they connected the oxygen tubing to the IV. Naturally, the oxygen went into the IV, immediately causing a large air embolism. Significant efforts to save the patient were made, but the patient ultimately passed away.

There are a few other similar examples (connecting tube feeding to an IV line or to a tracheostomy) that were all innocent and just the family member or loved one not wanting to bother the nurse, trying to take care of it themselves and ultimately causing irreparable damage. However, as you can see, this can have horrible repercussions! Please, please, please, make sure that if something becomes dislodged or disconnected that you let your nurse know immediately so that they can address it promptly.

The Heart Monitor

Not all patients will have a heart monitor, but many will. It is a device with wires and stickers that are attached to your chest to monitor your heart. Depending on whether you're in the intensive care unit or a regular nursing unit, the box may be next to your bed with long wires or in a pocket of your gown with much shorter wires, monitored in a different location.

We watch your heart all the time! However, if one of the stickers comes loose, we have to replace it to make sure we can see your heart rhythm. It's not a crisis if one becomes dislodged, but it must be promptly addressed. If the leads are not in place, we cannot see what your heart is doing from an electrical standpoint. A staff member will come in, peek under your gown, and see which lead needs to be replaced. The adhesive wears down after a few days, which is why we change them. They can leave a little bit of residue on your skin. This comes off with soap and water.

The Sequential Compression Devices (SCDs)

These are also called "leg squeezers" and are attached to both of your legs to prevent blood clots from forming. The longer you're in bed, the higher the risk is for blood clots to form. Therefore, we put these devices on your legs because you're not walking around like usual. They do not hurt. They just give a gentle squeeze, one leg at a time, to get the blood flowing!

If the doctor ordered them, you should wear them while you're in bed. They are only effective when they're being worn! If you're walking around, bathing, and so on, you do not need to wear them. However, when you get back in bed, they need to be put back on. This is something that is the last thing the nurse or nursing assistant will do when they get you back in bed, so please remind them to replace them if they've forgotten! With the hustle and bustle of getting all of the wires, lines, and tubes situated, these pumps can be forgotten.

Many patients will need some oxygen during their stay. Oxygen can be given in many different ways. We can give you a small amount through a clear tube that fits on your nose, or it can be given in a mask that goes on your face, or even a tube that goes down your throat. It all depends on the situation, and we like to make sure we are giving the least amount needed in the least aggressive way. Most times, the oxygen comes out of a fixture in the wall. When patients need to travel from their room to a procedure or a different room, oxygen tanks are used for the transfer.

Interventions and Essential Information

In addition to medical equipment, it is important that you are familiar with how various common interventions occur as well as how we educate you.

Fall Prevention

Every single facility in this country cares about preventing patients from falling. We do not want you to get injured while you are in the hospital; therefore we will do whatever we can to prevent this. This includes using all kinds of equipment to identify people who are more at risk for falling (like a patient who just had a knee surgery): signs on the hospital room door, wristbands, color-coded socks and gowns, and ensuring a staff member is with you or your loved one when walking or going to the restroom.

Procedures

There are many different kinds of procedures that can be performed during a hospital stay. Some of them are done in special areas of the hospital (sometimes called *procedural areas*; already mentioned on page 43 and page 49) or even in the operating room. There are also procedures that can be completed right in your hospital room (referred to as "bedside procedures"). If you or a loved one needs a procedure, the person performing the procedure will explain what is about to happen and where it is happening, along with the risks and benefits. Please, ask any and every question you have to make sure you understand everything. It is important to us that you understand.

Educational Materials

We like to make sure you know everything you need to know about your health and what's going on. However, we realize that while you're in the hospital it can be quite overwhelming to learn a lot of new things. It is important to us to know that you understand what is going on, which is why many facilities have educational materials available for patients and loved ones. While many times they are written materials, more and more facilities are creating different kinds of educational materials. Some examples of other educational resources include videos, interactive online resources, and audio education.

A Few Words about Food in the Hospital

Food is typically very important to patients and loved ones; understandably so! To be able to get patients food, the nursing and dietary staff must have an order from the physician saying that it is okay for the patient to eat. There may be reasons why you are not allowed to eat (typically related to a test, surgery, or procedure). Most nurses know this will be one of the first things patients will request (especially if the patient has been in the ED half the day!) so we are typically on top of it and make sure that if we are allowed to feed you, we are working on getting you food as quickly as possible.

Hospital Stay FAQs

1. *My loved one is in a private room with a bathroom. Is it okay if I use it?*

   Because of infection prevention and cross contamination, most prefer all visitors to use the public restrooms in the hospital (typically located in or near waiting rooms). Please make sure to ask the staff first.

2. *My loved one is in something called "isolation"—what does that mean?*

   If the health care team determines that you or your loved one has an organism that is resistant to antibiotics, a very contagious infection, or an immune system that cannot fight off infections, you or your loved one will be put on something called isolation precautions.

This means that the staff will typically wear additional protective gear when they are in your room. We want to make sure we are protecting you, but also protecting the other patients we are caring for as well. You will be educated specifically about the type of isolation, the reasoning, and what you need to do. We will put a sign on the door to let other staff know what they need to wear when in the room.

Isolation protective equipment (gowns, gloves, masks, etc.) are all one-time use items. Please do not keep your disposable gown and reuse it. We know it can be wasteful, but it is a safety concern to continue using the same one. This can be somewhat confusing for people, so please ask questions! Many hospitals will also provide written material explaining this to increase understanding.

3. *Can I bring them food from home?*

Ask the nurse if the food you would like to bring from home is within the prescribed diet and of the appropriate consistency. We want the patient to have food they enjoy and will eat. They need nourishment to heal, so if you have things at home that they prefer and they are appropriate within the constraints of the diet, go for it! Just make sure to *ask the nurse first.*

4. *Can I bring food to store for them?*

This can vary from unit to unit; however, most units do not have a large amount of refrigerator space or have one refrigerator for each room. Because we can't verify that the food was safely and properly prepared, as we can with the food that comes out of our kitchen, you may be required to sign a waiver.

We also do not put food in the unit fridge that has already been in the patient's room. If you've got a unit of 25 patients and 10 of them with various illnesses and diseases would like their leftover lunch in the fridge, that means there are containers from 10 different rooms with food patients have partially eaten all in the same small, contained area. Therefore, we typically do not allow food that has already been in the room into the communal fridge where we store extra juices, jellos, etc. If you or your loved one is on isolation, that food definitely cannot go in the fridge under any circumstances if it has been in the room already.

Medications in the Hospital

Your medications from home. When you're admitted to the hospital, someone will ask you for your list of home medications, better known as "meds." We put them into your chart and the doctor takes a look at them and decides which ones they want you to keep taking while in the hospital. While you may have been on a certain medication for years, it may not be good for you to take it during this admission, which is why the doctor reviews them.

While it is extremely important for us to maintain your normal home medication routine while you're in the hospital, not all medications that you normally take will be medically appropriate at that time.

Keep in mind, these are not necessarily permanent changes. Every single day, your health care team reviews your medications and makes changes as they are needed. They may add or remove medications. When you are discharged, they provide you with an updated list of changes and directions on what to stop taking, what to continue taking, and what to start taking so that you know beyond a shadow of a doubt exactly what to do.

Your new medications. The doctor will also look at why you are in the hospital and decide on which new medications to start giving you, if any. They will tell you what new medications you are to start taking, and you can always ask your nurse additional questions as needed. If it is something you would like printed information on, again, let your nurse know and he or she can get that for you. Bear in mind, though: the process of adding a medication—if not all aspects of in-hospital medication administration—can take longer than you might like. Please look at the box, *Adding New Medications*, to learn why.

If an emergency occurs and you or your loved one needs emergency medications, we readily have access to the necessary medications. In a code or emergency, we have a different process that we follow.

So yes: Adding a medication can take much longer than it seems like it should. However, you have three people double-checking that this medication is safe and appropriate for you: first the doctor, then the pharmacist, and finally the nurse. We can attempt to expedite this process as much as possible but these checks and balances are a very important aspect of patient safety.

Let's say your doctor has just come by to see you this morning and notes that your pain is not controlled by the medication you have been receiving. You're miserable.

▶ He or she decides to change your pain medication to something different. You're elated because you're willing to try anything at this point!

▶ After your physician leaves the room, you might expect your nurse to walk in soon with the new medication. However, this almost never happens quite that quickly. To some extent, it cannot, due to a process with checks and balances that must be followed. Here is a snapshot of it:

  ▶ After the physician leaves the room, a nurse will open your chart and add this medication.

  ▶ This sends an alert to a pharmacist who checks this medication with all of the other ones you're receiving (as well as your allergies) to make sure this medication is safe for you to receive.

  ▶ After the order is placed, the pharmacist gives their stamp of approval; the nurse will then be allowed to administer it.

  ▶ Once the nursing team receives the medication, they must verify it is correct and go through their process for appropriate administration.

Medication administration. Hospitals are required by law to keep every single medication under lock and key. We are legally required to do this, even if you bring in your home medications and want to keep them with you in your room. Also, the hospital typically prefers to use our medications but you can use your own if you would like as long as your doctor gives you the green light and communicates this with the nursing staff.

In order for you to be able to use your home meds, there is a process we must follow. We want to have an accurate record of what you are taking and when you are taking it, even if it is something you have been taking for years. It is very critical that we know and document all of the medications you receive while in the hospital. If you start to not do so well, one of the things we look at is what different medications you have received. If we have no idea what you've been taking, this presents a serious safety issue. Additionally, some of these home medications may interact with new medications. If we are unaware of what you are taking, we cannot prevent this and serious consequences can occur as a result.

Therefore, please make sure you give your nurse an accurate, up-to-date medication list, and send all medications home with a loved one unless you have the approval of your attending physician to take them while you're in the hospital. If the doctor does approve of this, the medication(s) must be locked up at all times. Please remember to get them before you're discharged.

Medication administration times. Many hospitals have designated times when nurses give medications. For example, if you tell the doctor you take all of your medications daily, they will all default for the nurse to give them to you at 9:00 a.m.. Your nurse will have a certain amount of time to give those medications (typically 30 to 60 minutes before and after the due time, depending on the unit). While you may have six pills due at 9:00 a.m., your nurse is also caring for other patients who have medications due at that time. This means that I, as the nurse, have from

8:00 a.m. to 9:59 a.m. to give all of my patients their 9:00 a.m. medications.

If you take your medications before breakfast, they will default to an earlier time (typically 6:30 a.m.). Or, if you take something three times per day, the times they typically default to are around 9:00 a.m., 1:00 p.m., and 5:00 p.m.

If you have a very specific time you would like your medications, please let your nurse know so they can adjust the times appropriately in your chart and also alert pharmacy. However, keep in mind that this cannot always be accommodated for various reasons established by the physician (new medications, conditions, etc.). There are examples of medications that must be given during a very tight timeframe and nurses are highly aware of these. They are few and far between, but exceptions to the rule do exist!

Scheduled medications and as-needed medications. When nurse opens your chart to see which medications to give you and when to administer them, they are separated into two groups: scheduled medications and as-needed medications. Scheduled meds have a due time and they alert the nurse to go in and give these meds at specific times.

As-needed medications show up to the nurse a little differently. We wait until we see, or you tell us, that you need them. Items in this category include medications for nausea, anxiety, seizures, pain, and fever, for example. Therefore, we have these medications readily available without having to call the physician for a nausea medication when you're actively throwing up.

Pain medications. In most cases, pain medications fall into the as-needed category. This means you need to alert the nurse when you feel you need some medication for pain. Nurses are routinely assessing pain; however, if you notice that you need medication, please let your nurse know. We typically like to see if other interventions (repositioning, heat/ice, calm environment, etc.) will work before administering these medications, but when you need them—you need them.

We strongly recommend that you do not wait until your pain is unbearable before you let you nurse know. Depending on the medication, it can take anywhere from 10 to 45 minutes for it to fully take effect. It is much easier to control your pain before it gets unbearable. If you wait until you can't take it anymore, the normal pain medication the doctor has for you may not be enough anymore, and if it was administered earlier it could have provided much better relief.

If you're hurting, we need to address it. It is harder for your body to heal if you're constantly in pain. You cannot rest, and you need rest to heal.

Pain management. There is also a common misconception about pain medication. I have had many patients believe that when they get the medication, it will take away all pain. This does not happen. It will help reduce the pain to a tolerable level, but pain medication does not relieve all pain and discomfort. The goal is to get it to a tolerable level to allow healing to occur. Getting up the first time after surgery will hurt. Having surgery in general hurts.

And unfortunately, a lot of things that we need to do in the hospital cause some degree of discomfort.

Pain *management* is the key, not pain *elimination*, for it is not possible to safely remove all pain every time. Pain medications are potent. They have many side effects. We don't like to use them if it's not necessary. One of the major side effects of many pain medications is something called respiratory depression. These medications can suppress your drive to breathe if given in high enough doses. If enough is given, they will stop you from breathing all together. Our goal is to use the least amount of pain medication in conjunction with other nonmedication-related therapies to achieve the best level of pain management.

Pain assessment. Nurses are required to regularly assess your pain level. We are also required to assess it more frequently if pain medications were given to you. The way we assess this is by asking you (if you're awake, alert, and able to answer questions appropriately) to rate your pain on a scale from 0 to 10. Zero means you have absolutely no pain and 10 means this is the most unbearable, unimaginable pain you've ever experienced in your life and it could not possibly get any worse. Again, we are required to ask you this question very frequently.

It is important to tell us exactly how your pain feels to you so we know how to treat it and promote optimal healing. I have provided you with an explanation of each number in the pain scale in Figure 1.

Subjective Pain Scale		
	0	No pain. Feeling perfectly normal.
Minor	1 **Very Mild**	Very light barely noticeable pain
Able to adapt to pain	2 **Discomforting**	Minor pain, like lightly pinching the fold of skin
	3 **Tolerable**	Very noticeable pain, like a doctor giving you an injection
Moderate	4 **Distressing**	Strong, deep pain, like an average toothache
Interferes with many activities	5 **Very Distressing**	Strong, deep, piercing pain, such as a sprained ankle
	6 **Intense**	Strong, deep, piercing pain, like several bee stings
Severe	7 **Very intense**	Comparable to an average migraine headache
	8 **Utterly Horrible**	Comparable to childbirth or a really bad migraine headache
Patient is disabled and unable to function independently	9 **Excruciating Unbearable**	Pain so intense you cannot tolerate it and demand pain killers
	10 **Unimaginable Unspeakable**	Pain so intense you will go unconscious shortly

FIGURE 1. A Subjective Pain Scale

SOME BASIC HOSPITAL PROCESSES: COMMUNICATION, TRANSFERS, DISCHARGES

As you have probably already learned, there is a lot of "hurry up and wait" that happens in the hospital. From getting to your room, to transferring to another room, to going home, things can take some time to happen.

Communication

As previously stated, most nursing units do not have a physician there 24-7. Methods of communication vary between facilities, but occasionally the physician or their support staff is not immediately available. Sometimes, they are in a procedure or surgery. Sometimes, they are in the middle of giving a patient very devastating news. And sometimes, they're right around the corner (if a nurse is lucky!). This is why it can take some time to get a hold of a physician.

Transfers

If the medical team comes by in the morning and decides that you will be transferring out of the intensive care unit to a regular nursing unit, the attending physician must review your chart, review all medications, and enter or discontinue orders and sign off on them. Furthermore, if multiple doctors are seeing you and the attending physician wants these other doctors to see you first before you're transferred to another room (typically if you are in intensive care or step-down and going to a regular room), we must also wait for them to round (again, their timing is unpredictable) and give us the green light.

Discharges

The same is true with being discharged. When your doctor comes by at 9:00 a.m. and lets you know that you will be going home this morning, it does not mean it is time to start packing up. That physician must sit down and document everything that is needed for your discharge. This includes medication changes, writing new prescriptions and facilitating getting them filled, follow-up appointments, and any new restrictions and recommendations. This information must be documented and in your chart, so the nurse can compile your discharge paperwork. We want to make sure everything is taken care of before you leave so you are well aware of all medication changes, follow-up appointments, any new restrictions, and any education provided to you during your stay.

SECTION 3

MY PERSONAL ADVICE: A NURSE SPEAKS TO YOU AND YOUR LOVED ONES

Working at the bedside for a while, I have seen many people go through routine situations, but I've also seen many different people from different life situations with different kinds (or lack) of support go through traumatic things. I've learned some things along the way, walking with patients and families through some of the toughest times in their lives. Being aware of these ahead of time can help you focus more on healing and getting home—which is really your primary goal as a patient.

This section covers these concerns:

▸ Promoting a healing environment

▸ Getting enough rest

▸ Establishing someone to speak on your behalf

▸ Advocating for yourself

▸ Knowing your code status

▸ A nurse's hardest work

▸ Dealing with information overload

▸ Coping as part of healing

▸ What the health care team needs from you

PROMOTE A HEALING ENVIRONMENT

There are a few things that go into making the environment you are in during your stay as healing as possible. Establishing a routine at the beginning of the day or night is essential. When your nurse comes by to introduce him or herself, make sure he or she is telling you what to expect for the next 12 hours. It would be helpful to know when someone will be coming by to take your vital signs or draw labs, who to expect will be coming by (for example, physical or occupational therapists) today, or if you will need to leave the unit for any reason. Knowing what to expect will allow you and your loved ones to get through each day more prepared and less anxious about what is to come.

Another aspect of a healing environment is controlling visitors. We know how valuable it can be to have the support of others during a hospital stay. As long as it is helpful to you and your healing, we want to encourage visitors. However, the line between visitors being helpful and tiring is not as obvious as one might think. Patients frequently feel the need to stay awake and visit with people who have taken the time to come see them in the hospital. This can cause patients to miss out on desperately needed rest. If you are getting overwhelmed with the amount of people coming to see you, let the staff know. We can always put a sign on your door and restrict visitors. We do not mind telling people to come back at a later time or to call first before visiting. Remember, your healing and your rest are what is most important!

Rest!

While you're in the hospital, it is important to sleep as much as possible during the night. People heal better when they are able not only to rest, but to rest at night and be awake during the day. This enables you to be as alert as possible during the day to allow you to work with your health care team, stay nourished, and promote your own healing.

If you are having trouble sleeping, let your nurse know. There are various things we can do to promote better sleep. From clustering our care so that there are minimal sleep interruptions to putting a sign on your door, providing medications, or blocking out light, we must make your rest a priority. If you need a nap during the day, we can let others know not to come in the room or to come back later.

Establish a Spokesperson

When someone becomes a patient in the hospital, the nurse will typically ask for the contact information of an emergency contact person. We want you to think of the one person you would want us to call if all of a sudden something happened. This should be a reliable person who can communicate to the rest of your loved ones for you when you are not able to do so.

We encourage you to identify this person so when changes and updates occur, the staff can call one person and they can communicate to the rest of your family or loved ones. This enables the entire health care team to make one phone call to get the message across, rather than making multiple calls and taking time away from being with you at the bedside.

It important that this person can be easily reached, that you trust this person with your health information, and that they are reliable and able to speak with the rest of your support system.

Advocate for Yourself

So what if things are not going well? What if you are not happy with your doctor, nurse, or physical therapist? How do you advocate for yourself or your loved ones to make sure you or they are getting the best care possible? There are a few ways to go about this.

The nurse manager. If you are unhappy with a member of your health care team, you can let your nurse know that you would like to speak with the nurse manager. They are typically available in person during business hours (Monday to Friday, 8:00 a.m. to 5:00 p.m.); however, this can vary. Even if the person or situation that you are not happy with did not involve a nurse, the nurse manager usually knows who to follow up with to get the problem addressed.

Patient relations. Many hospitals and facilities also have a department that addresses complaints, grievances, or issues that arise during a hospitalization. You can always ask the information desk if such a department, or similar one, is available at your facility. This department, if available, is one that is typically open during regular business hours

(Monday to Friday, 8:00 am to 5:00 pm) but this can also vary.

The alert line. Another resource available to advocate for yourself or a loved one is an alert line. This is a phone number that you can call, typically 24 hours a day, to report issues. This number is different for each facility. It can be located on informational posters, in your admission packet, or you can ask the information desk as well.

It is important that you advocate for yourself or your loved ones when something is happening or has happened that should not have occurred. Please tell us if an issue arises that needs to be addressed. We would love to correct and address this before you are discharged.

Know Your Code Status

Whenever someone is admitted to the hospital, the doctor will ask a very important question that the hospital is required to ask: your code status. We want to know exactly what you want us to do if you stop breathing (respiratory arrest), your heart stops (cardiac arrest), or both. We are required to ask you this question every single time you come to the hospital. We must know, beyond a shadow of a doubt, what you would want done in that situation. We must ask you (or someone who is authorized to make decisions on your behalf) every time because if you became unconscious, you could not answer this question.

This may be an easy question for many people to answer. You may not have any health issues and are not nearing the end of your life, and therefore you want everything done.

Or your religious, spiritual, or cultural beliefs will order this decision for you and you will know beyond a shadow of a doubt that you want everything done. Regardless of the situation, it is very important to understand what "everything" truly means.

When someone stops breathing ... We lay the patient flat and pull their head back as far as it goes and put an endotracheal tube (or some call it "breathing tube") down the throat. We attach it to a ventilator (or some call it a "breathing machine"), which will breathe for the patient.

When someone's heart stops ... The first thing we do is initiate cardiopulmonary resuscitation (CPR). Basically, the heart has stopped beating and therefore is not supplying blood to the body. So the brain, lungs, kidneys, and everything else are not getting blood. When things don't get blood, they die quickly. Therefore, a staff member will stand above the bed and forcefully push down on the chest to pump the heart. This is a traumatic but necessary task. Force is necessary because the rib cage is protecting the heart. Many times, multiple ribs are broken so that the heart can be manually pumped effectively. In such cases, broken ribs are an indication of doing it right. Remember, we're trying to get blood to the brain, lungs, and other organs to make sure their cells don't die, so broken ribs are the least of our worries right now.

While this is occurring, another person is putting a defibrillator on the patient. In movies and on television, it is typically portrayed as someone coming at the patient with paddles, ready to shock. These are outdated; most hospital use adhesive pads that we stick to the patient's chest. This device is able to interpret the heart rhythm for the nurses and physicians at the bedside so we know what to do next. Depending on what the heart is doing, we can give medications or we can provide electric current to shock the heart back to a nonlethal rhythm. We cannot just give medications for every situation; many times an electrical shock is needed.

When any of this happens, "doing everything" can encompass more things, but these are the main interventions that will occur for someone who has stopped breathing or whose heart has stopped.

As you can imagine, this is a pretty traumatic process for the patient, their loved ones, and even the health care providers who address these situations every day. It is important to know if this is what you want done to yourself and if this is what your loved ones want for themselves, should the situation present itself.

To clarify, if you or your loved ones want "everything done"—this includes the above-mentioned interventions and means you will be classified as a "full code."

If this sounds like something you do not want for yourself, or something you think your loved one might not want, please let your health care team know. If you have a terminal diagnosis, are of advanced age, etc., you may want to die a natural death. This is called a "Do Not Resuscitate" order or "DNR" order. A DNR means that if you stop breathing or your heart stops, we provide you with comfort measures and allow you to pass. No breathing tube, no broken ribs, no electrical shock.

Please know that if you decide to be a DNR, we need to make sure everyone caring for you knows this. Typically, hospitals have a policy requiring all patients who want to be a DNR to wear a bracelet that indicates this. We do this so that no matter where you are in the hospital, whether you went to radiology for an x-ray or are transferring units, everyone can see that if your heart stops on the elevator, we are not to call the code team and immediately start CPR. (Yes, people do code in elevators!) While it may be emotionally difficult to see that wristband or label, it is essential to ensure your wishes are followed, no matter the circumstance or location within our walls.

Please anticipate this question from the doctor when you are coming into the hospital. Also, we do know that it is not always as black and white as I just described it above. Maybe you are okay with getting the breathing tube, but you do not want someone performing CPR. We can talk about those specifics and make sure your wishes are followed.

As a nurse who has seen this situation play out many times before, I can tell you that it is much easier on the loved ones to never insert the breathing tube than have to face the decision of removing it. Taking things away is much more difficult than not getting them in the first place. This is why talking about this and making this decision beforehand is so important. It's much easier to think about, process, and consider everything when it's not in the midst of a chaotic emergency.

Some loved ones feel that they must do everything in every situation, or else it means they do not love the patient or want them to be alive. This could not be further from the truth.

Sometimes, allowing someone to die a natural peaceful death—despite how emotionally painful it may be—is the most loving and caring thing we can do. Sometimes, out of this feeling of obligation we —members of the health care team and the family and other decision-makers—rob patients of the ability to exit this world in a peaceful and comfortable manner.

No one can make this decision for you. As an experienced health care provider I can only share with you the knowledge that I have acquired, having seen this situation occur many times. I want you and your loved ones to make informed decisions about the end of your life and how you ideally want it to look and feel.

THE HARDEST WORK THAT NURSES DO

Without a doubt, the absolute hardest thing to watch as a nurse is when a patient is dying but the family or support system cannot come to terms with that. The patient is continually put through needless and painful rounds of test after test, procedure after procedure, and day after day in the hospital. When the family is not around, the patient is trying to communicate that they want to die. They want to be allowed to pass.

You will hear some family members say, "He/she would never have wanted this," but the *health care power of attorney* (HCPOA) or main decision-makers can't see through their pain to make the right decision for their loved one. If the patient's HCPOA or next of kin decides this is what they want, we must follow it, even if the patient appears to not want it. The patient must be of sound mind to make that decision. So, if someone is in and out of consciousness or lucidity, they legally cannot make that decision for themselves; the health care team must go to the HCPOA or next of kin. Unfortunately, some patients at the end of their life are not of sound mind and cannot make that decision.

> **Health care power of attorney (HCPOA):** A legal document that gives a person (Person 2), who is selected by an individual who is a patient-to-be (Person 1), the power to make medical decisions when Person-1 is no longer able to do so. This document is active only when Person-1 is unable to make personal decisions or even to communicate.

This is a terrible and painful way to exit this world. And I've seen it more times than I can count. It is all too common.

Believe it or not, this is so difficult to endure that health care employees experience post-traumatic stress disorder and emotional distress from these and similar situations. In fact, many hospitals even have their own counseling programs for their employees because it can be so distressing.

It is essential, no matter how old you are, to think about what will be important to you when the time comes for your life to end. In an ideal situation, what do you want that to look and feel like? What's important to you physically, emotionally, and spiritually? It is important for every single person on this earth to think about that, decide what they want, and communicate that clearly to their loved ones.

This is not an easy thing to discuss, but it could not be more important.

The last thing anyone should have to go through is never discussing this in your life and then suddenly your worst nightmare occurs and you are faced with making a major decision for someone else, never having spoken about it before. Please, don't wait until you're in the situation. Do it now, when you're thinking about your life and the ones you love around you. Talking about it and making your wishes clearly known will facilitate their grieving your peaceful passing.

The experience will be so different if this is done beforehand. Families who know beyond a shadow of a doubt exactly what their loved one would have wanted are able to make decisions sooner, prevent suffering, and allow themselves the ability to grieve and be at peace. If they don't know for sure exactly what to do, they are going through emotional distress trying to figure out what their loved one would have wanted, hoping it was the right decision, and then living with that decision the rest of their lives.

So, please have this conversation now. Please figure out what you want, what is important to you, and *who* is important to you. If your loved ones are asked to make the decision between you dying or living in a nursing home for the rest of your life, they need to be empowered to answer with confidence.

So how do you go about doing this? It is not an easy thing to talk about, especially if this is a topic you've never talked about with anyone.

The first step is to figure out what you want. Think about what is and is not important to you. If living in a nursing home, dependent on others to care for you or death were your only options, what would you want? If you needed a machine to help you breathe and food given to you through a tube, and were not able to take care of yourself, would that be okay? There is no one answer for everyone. It is all about what is right for you.

Next, identify someone you love and whose judgment you trust. This may not be the most obvious person. It may not be your spouse, one of your parents, or your children. A person who you trust to put your desires and needs above their own. A person who can think through their own emotion and pain and do the right thing.

Then, ask a very, very important question: "If I can't make my own medical decisions at some point, will you make them for me?" Outline with this person what you do and do not want. Talk to your other loved ones and make sure they know. If there are family members who would be upset if you did not pick them, let them know that you needed to pick someone who would be able to make this decision even when walking through his or her worst nightmare. Someone who could see through his or her own pain and do what you asked.

As mentioned earlier: many people create a legal document called a health care power of attorney (HCPOA). Doing this is always a good idea. An HCPOA can be completed in most hospitals or even online. Legal requirements vary from state to state, as some states require them to be notarized and others do not. This document specifies a person to make decisions for you.

You can also complete a living will. This document says what you would want done if certain situations presented themselves. Both are very helpful in tough situations. Also, if you are moving to a new state, make sure you give a copy to your new health care provider and make sure it meets all of their requirements. Ask a member of your health care team if you're interested in setting one up while you're in the hospital. Please remember, people must be of sound mind to sign these documents.

Please do not make the mistake of only talking to one person, designating a health care power of attorney and making a living will, and then keeping it to yourself. While this document is important, it is much more important that all of your loved ones and your entire support system are aware of your wishes. This prevents arguing, anguish, and disagreements during tough times.

> **Living will:** A legal document that outlines the specific medical treatments that someone either wants or doesn't want for when a person is unable to make such decisions. Typically, it states clearly the desire for certain medical scenarios; for example, "I do not want a breathing tube if there is no possibility of a normal life," or "I do want a breathing tube, even if there is no possibility of a normal life."

Disagreements and arguments about what to do in an intensive care waiting room while, say, Dad is on a ventilator with pneumonia and minimal brain function are dreadful. Conversations about death are essential, and if you've never openly talked about it with your family, chances are they haven't really had to realistically think about you dying, let alone what to do.

Prayerfully, you will never need this document, the situation will never present itself, and your loved one will never be faced with this decision. But in the event that it does occur, you and your loved ones will know exactly what to do, trusting and knowing they did the right thing.

> **PATIENT TIP!** Write things down. It can be hard to remember which doctor said what, the name of the new medications, what exercises the physical therapist recommended, etc. Write these important pieces of information down so hat you don't forget. I have provided space in the back for you to take notes.

DEALING WITH INFORMATION OVERLOAD

During your stay you will hear a lot of new information. It can be difficult to remember new medications, diagnoses, etc., especially if you're already having trouble understanding what is already going on! If you need written information, please ask. Many nursing units have educational materials that they can easily provide.

Please know that we are aware that you and your loved ones are getting a lot of new information in a short amount of time. Your entire health care team is aware that many medical conditions are very complex and it may take having it explained to you a few times before you really understand what's going on. It is understandable if you need things explained to you or your loved ones a few times before it really sinks in. Please do not think you're being annoying when you're asking for us to explain exactly what is going on and what our goals are again. It is essential for you to understand this information and it can be explained as many times as necessary to make sure you know what is going on.

COPING AS A PART OF HEALING

Sometimes, getting back to normal takes a lot of work. It can take working with all of the therapy service team members multiple times a day, even when you're tired or it hurts. It means taking medications that taste bad, but what they do for your healing is so important that it's worth it. It can mean asking your visitors to step out so you can rest. It can mean getting up and walking around the unit multiple times a day, even if you really don't want to.

We know that healing, facing new challenges and diagnoses, and being in the hospital, especially for unplanned incidents, is stressful. We know that many people have different kinds of coping mechanisms that they use at home that can't be used in the hospital. Alcohol, smoking, food, various drugs, caffeine, and other things are frequently used by patients and loved ones outside of the hospital. If you're having trouble coping, please let us know. Maybe there is some resource, medication, therapy, etc., that we can utilize to help ease your healing. We want you to heal. We want you to feel safe. We want you to be healthy. Please communicate with us if you are having a tough time.

WHAT THE HEALTH CARE TEAM NEEDS FROM YOU

I've talked a lot about what your health care team does and what you should expect of them. It is important to also know what the team expects from you, as the patient, and from your support system.

You are the reason we are here. You are the reason we come to work every day. We enjoy taking care of people and providing the best care to help you get back to your life. We want you to care about your health. We want you to care about doing the best you possibly can for yourself. We want to enable this. Please let us know how we can support and empower you in this.

You are worth working for your health. You are worth all of this work to get better. We want you to know and believe that.

SECTION 4
DURING YOUR STAY: YOUR INFORMATION!

When you're in a hospital, new information is constantly being thrown at you. It can feel like you're trying to drink from a fire hose! Below are some recommendations of notes to take during your stay, especially if you have multiple physicians or it's an extended stay. You can look at it later with fresh eyes, after a shower or rest, and allow the information to really sink in.

WHAT KINDS OF INFORMATION?

It's been my experience that these following categories will capture most of the information you'll need to have close at hand…. But make sure to add anything you or loved ones think useful, may easily forget, or will need to communicate to the rest of the support system.

> **Write down who is who.** Doctors take vacations or switch call days sometimes, so you don't always know who is coming into the room every day unless they tell you who they are. Nurses change from shift to shift and also take vacations and days off. Write down each of their names and what kind of doctor or nurse she or he is they are as well as other members of the health care team whom you would like to remember.

Write down important things your health care team tells you. When you have multiple doctors from different service lines telling you different things, it can be hard to put the big clinical picture together. Many times the doctors don't actually talk to each other; they write notes in your chart for the other doctors to read. You and your loved ones are the common denominator. So, if you find an inconsistency with what one physician, nurse, or other member of the health care team is saying compared to another, make sure you ask them about it and let them know it is different from what someone else has told you. It really helps to know who is who, and who is saying what—so don't be afraid to ask to make sure that you are firm in understanding the whole picture!

Write down people who you really appreciated. Whether they are from housekeeping, the pharmacy, the nursing unit or any of the physicians, write down people who went the extra mile for you. Occasionally, management will round and check on you, or you may have another opportunity at some point to recognize them for giving that extra special effort. It can be really hard days later to remember names, but you may want to recognize all the hard work done by hospital staff members!

Write down questions as you think of them and answers as you receive them. You think you won't forget questions as they come up, but it never fails that they leave your mind when the doctor is rounding! As soon as you think of a question, write it down. Once you receive the answer, write that down as well. If you are not sure why something is occurring (like a test, procedure, or medication), write down that you need it explained further so the next time your nurse or doctor comes by, you can ask and write down the answer. It is important to write down the question as well as the answer. When your concern gets clarified, it may make sense at that time, but you may forget later on.

Write down your emergency contacts. Things can get a little hazy when you're in a new environment like the hospital, and when you've had medications. This can be a great reference if you need someone to call a loved one for you, or if you want to call later yourself.

Important Questions to Ask as You Begin Your Stay

It is essential to know the answers to the below questions so that you can get better and get home as quickly as possible, and so that you are able to make informed decisions at every step of the way. If you don't know the answers to these questions, ask your nurse. Your nurse will most likely know the answer and if he or she does not know the answer, they know who to contact to obtain the answer for you.

▶ Why am I here?

▶ What medications am I taking? What medications are added or discontinued during my stay?

▶ What is the overall plan to get me home?

- What is everyone's overall goal for me? Every day, each member of the health care team (i.e., everyone) should have a goal in mind for you.

- What are my personal goals for my stay? What do I want and need to accomplish?

- What do I need to be thinking about for discharge? (For example, transportation, support, medications.)

- Do I have any financial concerns?

- Is there anything I need to take care of at home? (Such as: pet care, bills, family responsibilities, etc.) Who can help me take care of this?

- Any other questions that might occur to you.

Please use the last few pages of this book for you and your loved ones to make notes for yourself about your stay. Stay informed, ask good questions, and welcome to the team! It truly is a privilege and an honor to care for you.

MY HOSPITAL STAY

The next 16 pages are for you or loved ones for note-taking during your stay. If you don't like writing in books, you can photocopy these pages. Pages 89 through 98 have been created to handle your note taking for a single-day inpatient stay. If your stay extends into another day, you can use pages 99–104. Beyond that: photocopying!

My Name:

Admission date:

Discharge date:

Code status:

Nursing unit(s) and room number(s):

My emergency contacts, their relationship to
me, and their contact information:

Allergies:

My medications coming into the hospital:

My personal goals for my hospital stay:

My health care team's goals for me during my stay:

My new medications during my stay:

My personal goals today:

My health care team's goals for me today:

What is your name and from which service (specialty)? For example,
Dr. Smith with Cardiology, Dr. Jones with Nephrology, etc.

What has changed since the last time we spoke?

What are your plans and goals for me today?

What progress do you hope to see between
now and the next time you round?

Is there anything I can be doing to meet my goals?

What is your name?

What are nursing's plan and goals for me this shift?

How do I get a hold of you?

Is a nursing assistant working with me today? If so, her/his name and how do I get a hold of her/him?

Is there anything I can be doing to meet my goals?

What is your name?

What are nursing's plan and goals for me this shift?

How do I get a hold of you?

Is a nursing assistant working with me today? If so, her/his name and how do I get a hold of her/him?

Is there anything I can be doing to meet my goals?

Name, title, and department:

What role do you play on my health care team?

What are your plans and goals for me?

Is there anything I can be doing to meet these goals?

How often will you or a colleague be seeing me?

GOING HOME

Discharge date:

Who is taking me home? Will they be able to pick me up and bring me home upon discharge?

My new medications for home:

Where and when will I pick up my new medications? Will I pick them up from my pharmacy or get them at the hospital pharmacy before leaving?

Do I understand all of my new medications and when to take the next dose?

Who will be helping me at home? Do they need to be present during my discharge instructions from my nurse?

Do I know when and with whom I need to follow up and their contact information?

Am I concerned about going home at all? What questions do I have that must be answered before I am discharged?

When I have questions or concerns about my hospitalizations, or new symptoms arise, who do I call:

• During office hours:

• After business hours:

OTHER QUESTIONS FOR MY HEALTH CARE TEAM
+ NOTES

Doctors Taking Care of Me and Their Specialty (Daily)

Nurses Taking Care of Me (Each Shift): Shift One

Nurses Taking Care of Me (Each Shift): Shift Two

Other Hospital Staff Taking Care of Me (Daily)

OTHER QUESTIONS FOR MY HEALTH CARE TEAM
+ NOTES

INDEX

A

activities of daily living
(ADLs) 10, 27
admission into a hospital 54–58
advanced practice registered
nurses (APRNs) 5–6
certified nurse midwives
(CNMs) 5–6
certified registered nurse
anesthetists (CRNAs) 5
clinical nurse specialists
(CNSs) 5
nurse practitioners (NPs) 5
advocacy 72–73
for patient 72–73
American Nurses Credentialing
Center (ANCC) 5
associate's degree in nursing
(ADN) 2, 4
attending physicians 14

B

Bachelor of Science in Nursing
(BSN) ix, 4–5
bedside reporting 8
breathing machines 29
breathing stopped and code
status 73

C

call bells 50–51
cardiac arrest 73–77
cardiopulmonary resuscitation
(CPR) 74–75, 76
care coodrinators 35–36

care coordination. *See* case
managers
case managers 35–36
certified nurse midwives
(CNMs) 5–6
certified nurses 3–4
certified nursing assistants
(CNAs) 10
certified registered nurse
anesthetists (CRNAs) 5, 17
chaplains 33–34
charge nurse 11–12
defined 2
clinical nurse specialists (CNSs) 5
code status 73–77
Do Not Resuscitate (DNR)
order 75
full code 75
communication 66
consulting physicians 15–22
medical specialties 17–20
allergy and immunology 17
anesthesiology 17
dermatology 17
emergency medicine 17–18
family medicine 18
hospitalists 18
internal medicine 18–19
neurology 18
pathology 19
pediatrics 19
physical medicine and
rehabilitation 19
psychiatry and mental
health 19
radiology 19
surgical specialties 20–22

occupational therapists 27
physical therapists 26–27
respiratory therapists 31
transfers 66–67
tube feeding 33, 31